Emotion-Focused Counselling in Action

SAGE Counselling in Action

Series Editor: WINDY DRYDEN

SAGE Counselling in Action is a bestselling series of short, practical introductions designed for students and trainees. Covering theory and practice, the books are core texts for many courses, both in counselling and other professions such as nursing, social work and teaching. Books in the series include:

Andrew Reeves and Tim Bond
Standards and Ethics for Counselling in Action, Fifth Edition

Robert Elliott and Leslie Greenberg
Emotion-Focused Counselling in Action

Megan Rose Stafford and Tim Bond
Counselling Skills in Action, Fourth Edition

Michael Jacobs
Psychodynamic Counselling in Action, Fifth Edition

Peter Trower, Jason Jones and Windy Dryden
Cognitive Behavioural Counselling in Action, Third Edition

Dave Mearns and Brian Thorne with John McLeod
Person-Centred Counselling in Action, Fourth Edition

Petrūska Clarkson updated by Simon Cavicchia
Gestalt Counselling in Action, Fourth Edition

Ian Stewart
Transactional Analysis Counselling in Action, Fourth Edition

Diana Whitmore
Psychosynthesis Counselling in Action, Fourth Edition

Windy Dryden and Andrew Reeves
Key Issues for Counselling in Action, Second Edition

Windy Dryden
Rational Emotive Behavioural Counselling in Action, Third Edition

Patricia D'Ardenne and Aruna Mahtini
Transcultural Counselling in Action, Second Edition

Emotion-Focused Counselling in Action

Robert Elliott & Leslie Greenberg

SAGE Counselling in Action
Series Editor Windy Dryden

§SAGE

Los Angeles | London | New Delhi
Singapore | Washington DC | Melbourne

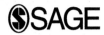

Los Angeles | London | New Delhi
Singapore | Washington DC | Melbourne

SAGE Publications Ltd
1 Oliver's Yard
55 City Road
London EC1Y 1SP

SAGE Publications Inc.
2455 Teller Road
Thousand Oaks, California 91320

SAGE Publications India Pvt Ltd
B 1/I 1 Mohan Cooperative Industrial Area
Mathura Road
New Delhi 110 044

SAGE Publications Asia-Pacific Pte Ltd
3 Church Street
#10-04 Samsung Hub
Singapore 049483

Editor: Susannah Trefgarne
Assistant editor: Ruth Lilly
Production editor: Manmeet Kaur Tura
Copyeditor: Sarah Bury
Proofreader: Christine Bitten
Indexer: David Rudeforth
Marketing manager: Dilhara Attygalle
Cover design: Naomi Robinson
Typeset by: C&M Digitals (P) Ltd, Chennai, India
Printed in the UK

Library of Congress Control Number: 2020947337

British Library Cataloguing in Publication data

A catalogue record for this book is available from the British Library

ISBN 978-1-4462-5723-4
ISBN 978-1-4462-5724-1 (pbk)

At SAGE we take sustainability seriously. Most of our products are printed in the UK using responsibly sourced papers and boards. When we print overseas we ensure sustainable papers are used as measured by the PREPS grading system. We undertake an annual audit to monitor our sustainability.

To all our students, colleagues and clients who have supported the development of an emotion-focused approach.

Contents

List of Figures and Tables

Figure

Tables

About the Authors

Robert Elliott is Professor of Counselling at the University of Strathclyde. He received his doctorate in clinical psychology from the University of California, Los Angeles, and is Professor Emeritus of psychology at the University of Toledo (Ohio). In collaboration with Leslie Greenberg and Laura Rice, he developed Emotion-Focused Therapy (EFT). He delivers EFT training internationally and within the UK. He serves on the board of the International Society for Emotion-Focused Therapy. He is co-author of *Facilitating emotional change* (1993), *Learning emotion-focused psychotherapy* (2004), *Research methods in clinical psychology* (2015), and *Essentials of descriptive-interpretive qualitative research* (2021), as well as more than 170 journal articles and book chapters. He is past president of the Society for Psychotherapy Research, and previously co-edited the journals *Psychotherapy Research* and *Person-Centered and Experiential Psychotherapies*. He is a fellow in the divisions of Clinical Psychology, Psychotherapy, and Humanistic Psychology of the American Psychological Association. He is a past recipient of the Distinguished Research Career Award of the Society for Psychotherapy Research, and the Carl Rogers Award from the Division of Humanistic Psychology of the American Psychological Association. He enjoys running, science fiction, poetry, and all kinds of music.

Leslie Greenberg is Distinguished Research Professor Emeritus of Psychology at York University in Toronto. Born in South Africa and originally an engineer, where he came to believe in tacit knowledge, that we know more than we can say, he switched to psychology in 1970 and trained in both Person-centred and Gestalt therapy. He has been engaged in psychotherapy research for over 40 years. He has authored major texts on Emotion-Focused Therapy, starting with the first books on *Emotion in psychotherapy* (1986) and *Emotionally focused therapy for couples* (1988) and *Facilitating emotional change*, with Laura Rice and Robert Elliott (1993). More recent books are *Emotion-focused therapy* (2015), *Case formulation in emotion-focused therapy* with Rhonda Goldman (2015), *Emotion-focused therapy of forgiveness and letting go* (2019) with Catalina Woldarsky, and *Emotion-focused therapy of generalized anxiety* (2017) with Jeanne Watson. He has received both the Early Career and the Distinguished Research Career awards of the International Society for Psychotherapy Research as well as the Carl Rogers and the Distinguished Professional Contribution to Applied Research awards of the American Psychological Association. He has also received the Canadian Psychological Association Professional Award for distinguished contributions to Psychology as a profession. He is a past President of the Society for Psychotherapy Research. He now spends most of his time training people nationally and internationally in Emotion-Focused Therapy. He has two adult children and two grandchildren and all live in Toronto.

Preface

Emotion-Focused Counselling (EFC) is a contemporary humanistic-experiential form of counselling that combines what we see as the best of Carl Rogers' person-centred approach and Fritz Perls' Gestalt therapy. We are humanists first, subscribing to a set of values that focus on the positive potential of people, the value of lived experience, the importance of cherishing diversity in ourselves and others, and the importance of treating others as equal in value and dignity to ourselves. These values have never been more important than they are today, as we find ourselves in the midst of both a pandemic and a worldwide outcry against various forms of inequality and authoritarianism. We believe that EFC has particular relevance to the present moment in which we find ourselves. Its theory of emotion points to the fundamental commonality among all human beings, while also explaining the basis of implicit bias and various forms of prejudice as maladaptive and secondary emotion processes and how these can be changed; its evidence base gives it credibility in an age of evidence-based practice; and its range of emotion theory concepts and tasks enable it to meet the diverse needs of people from diverse cultures and life situations.

The person-centred approach, in its contemporary incarnation as Person-Centred-Experiential (PCE) counselling, is one of the major theoretical approaches to counselling in the UK, and so in this book we emphasize our person-centred roots and the connection between EFC and PCE counselling. After all, our first counselling trainers (Jerry Goodman and Laura Rice) were students of Carl Rogers and we still find its relational stance to be most consistent with our values and practice. To that we've added the active task focus of Gestalt therapy, in which Les trained at the Gestalt Institute of Canada, in particular for its focus on the here and now and its use of experiments and enactments of parts of self and important others. Add a sprinkling of existential therapy, wrap it in emotion theory, and voila! Emotion-Focused Counselling.

A note on the case material in this book. Most of the client material used here comes from two clients, one seen by Robert and the other seen by a student of Les supervised by him. Each client gave their permission for material from their counselling to be used for research and teaching purposes, and we have also changed some of their details to protect their identity and edited the transcripts of their sessions for brevity and clarity.

This book may be relatively short, but it has taken almost 15 years to find the space in our busy lives to produce it and nearly 50 years of our own personal, professional, and scientific development to get here. We thank our students and clients for their inspiration over this time. We particularly thank Susannah Trefgarne for her patience and persistence over the long gestation of this book, and our reviewers and advance reader, Christina Michael.

Robert & Les (August 2020)

1

Emotion-Focused Counselling and the Person-Centred-Experiential Approach

---

Chapter Outline

Introducing Emotion-Focused Counselling

What is Emotion-Focused Counselling?

The Evolution of Emotion-Focused Counselling

Practising Emotion-Focused Counselling: Pre-flight Checklist

Emotion-Focused Counselling Practice Principles

Common Concerns Raised about Emotion-Focused Counselling

The Evidence on the Effectiveness of the Approach

Suggestions for Helping with the Process of Learning

Introducing Our Two Case Examples

Further Exploration

Introducing Emotion-Focused Counselling

Robert's new client is sitting nervously in the waiting room when he goes out to meet her at the beginning of their first session. 'Bethany?' he says, tentatively. She rises; they shake hands, exchange greetings, and he ushers her into the therapy room, letting her pick which of the three chairs she wants to sit in. She sits down a bit awkwardly, wrapping herself into a kind of human pretzel by twisting her arms and legs over each other.

Robert is struck by her body position, feeling it as a kind of expression of her fear of others, and finds himself resonating with a sense of her fearful uncertainty about what will happen in the work they are about to start. He deliberately fusses a bit with the recording equipment and papers to give her a bit of space.

Bethany:	Where are you from?
Robert (realizing that she is trying to take the focus off herself, he smiles to himself):	So you want to know a bit about me. From my accent you'll be able to tell that I'm American, but I've been in Scotland for 10 years. (He sits down, turns on the recorder.) I've been doing counselling for a while, but that doesn't stop me from being a bit nervous when I start with a new person. I wonder what you're experiencing, right now, as we start counselling?
Bethany (hesitantly):	Er… kind of, er, apprehensive?

This gives them a starting point, and they go into a small Focusing task by asking her a series of exploratory questions that help her explore where and how in her body she feels this 'apprehensive' (a tightness in her upper chest and throat), what it's about (meeting new people), what word or image might capture this feeling ('a bomb'), and what it is telling her ('to leave': the room or the subject of how she feels). After this, he offers a brief piece of *experiential teaching*, explaining that fear and anxiety are part of our evolutionary heritage, and are useful for warning us about dangers and can help us prepare for dealing with them.

This way of starting therapy with a highly socially anxious client doesn't fit the stereotype of person-centred counselling. First, there are three chairs (because in later sessions they will need the extra chair for two chair and empty chair work; see Chapters 6 and 7); second, the therapist asks a series of questions, clearly directing the process (we prefer to call this *process guiding*); third, there is a little bit of *Focusing* (borrowed and adapted from Gendlin, 1981; see Chapter 5), an example of what is called a *task* in the emotion-focused approach, where they collaborate with the client in working in a particular way with a particular issue in the session. Finally, they even talk a little bit about emotion theory with the client (see Chapter 2), which is part of creating a *working alliance* in EFC (see Chapter 4).

At the same time, the therapist in this vignette is clearly offering the Person-Centred therapeutic conditions (Rogers, 1957). Empathy is most clearly present, including the therapist using his body to *empathically resonate* with the client's anxiety at their first encounter, but he also offers a *process reflection* ('So you want to know a bit about me'), and carefully reflects each bit of the client's experience during the Focusing as well as offering *empathic conjectures* about as-yet unspoken aspects of what the client may be experiencing. *Genuineness* or *congruence* is easy to see as well, for example in the *process disclosure* that like the client he too is anxious about meeting a new person, but also in the evident pleasure he takes in beginning to learn about the client's experience of starting therapy. This gentle, warm curiosity is also evidence of *unconditional positive regard* (UPR), as is his nondefensive acceptance of the client's attempt to shift the conversational burden onto him by asking him about himself and her confession that her apprehension is telling her to leave the counselling room. Above all, this little bit of therapeutic work conveys the therapist's foremost desire to enter into a relationship with this client, to shift the power balance away from himself, and to encounter her as a fellow human being.

You will have also noticed that we've used quite a bit of EFC jargon to talk about what is going on in the session. EFC is big on *process differentiation*, that is to say, in this approach we like to carefully distinguish different aspects of things (what the client and counsellor do in the session, different aspects and kinds of emotions, different kinds and stages of emotion work, and so on). We don't do this to make ourselves powerful experts who speak a special, difficult-to-understand language to impress people with how clever we are. On the contrary, we want to honour the cleverness of our clients, to reveal and bring out their unstated expertise. EFC uses lots of different terms for what the client and counsellor do and experience in the session to help counsellors be as responsive as possible to their clients.

In this book, we want to introduce you to the Emotion-Focused approach to counselling or psychotherapy. In the relatively brief space we have here, our goal is to present this approach in a clear, accessible way. We start here in this chapter by describing where the approach came from and providing an overview of its essential features. In the following chapters we present its underpinning theory of emotion (Chapters 2 and 3), its opening phase of relationship building and beginning the work of therapy (Chapter 4), its early and late working phases of using therapeutic tasks to help clients deepen and transform their stuck emotions (Chapters 5–8), and the ending phase of consolidating and bringing therapy to a close (Chapter 9). We conclude with a discussion of how you can go further with this approach, should you be inspired to do so (as we hope you will be!) (Chapter 10).

What is Emotion-Focused Counselling?

As the initial case example shows, Emotion-Focused Counselling (EFC), more commonly called Emotion-Focused Therapy (EFT), is a contemporary form of the *Person-Centred-Experiential (PCE) Approach*, and has as its most important sources Carl Rogers' and Fritz Perls' deeply humanistic visions of therapeutic change.

EFC is, as its label clearly says, *focused on emotion*, not emotion as an abstract entity, but emotions in all their concrete, embodied, messy confusion, including the range of our immediate, moment-by-moment emotions: the small, subtle ones as well as the big, powerful ones. Emotions fill our lives and give them meaning, flavour and direction. Without emotions, we strongly believe, life would be colourless, empty and without meaning.

EFC is a *humanistic* therapy, embodying centuries of humanistic values, such as authenticity, growth, self-determination, creativity, equality, and pluralism. These values have often put humanists at odds with authority and power structures, but in their hearts humanistic therapists want to help their clients live fuller, more meaningful lives of mature interdependence with others (Fairburn, 1952; Lewin, 1948).

EFC is an *integrative* approach, pulling together key forms of practice from across the humanistic therapy tradition, including not just the Person-Centred approach of Carl Rogers (1951, 1957, 1961), but also the dramatic, active approach of Psychodrama (Moreno & Moreno, 1959) and Perls' Gestalt therapy (1969; Perls, Hefferline, & Goodman, 1951). Other key humanistic influences are existential psychotherapy (e.g., Schneider & Krug, 2017), with its focus on what is most important in lived, human existence, and narrative therapy (Angus & Greenberg, 2011), which recognizes the key role of context, story, and story-telling for human beings.

Finally, EFC is *evidence-based*. As we explain later in this chapter, it emerged out of the careful study of how clients change in sessions and is supported by a strong and growing base of outcome research, both quantitative and qualitative (see reviews by Elliott, Watson, Greenberg, Timulak, & Freire, 2013; Elliott, Watson, Timulak, & Sharbanee, in press; Timulak, Iwakabe, & Elliott, 2019). This also includes the development of a wide range of useful research tools that can be used to support practice and evidence-based models of how clients accomplish specific kinds of work in sessions (see Chapter 10).

The Evolution of Emotion-Focused Counselling

As noted, the roots of EFC lie firmly in the western humanistic tradition, which goes back ultimately to various ancient Greek philosophers (e.g., Aristotle, Epicurus), who focused their attention on humans rather than the gods and who advocated using human reason to understand the world. During the eighteenth-century Enlightenment period this tradition sought first to free itself from religious authority, then in the nineteenth century emphasized freedom and emotion as part of the Romantic movement (Coates, White, & Schapiro, 1966). In the twentieth century, humanism took the form of phenomenology, the study of direct human experience (Spinelli, 1989), and existentialism, which grounded itself in the fundamental human experiences of freedom, death, loneliness, responsibility, and meaning (Schneider & Krug, 2017; Yalom, 1980).

Humanistic psychotherapies expanded rapidly in the 1950s and 1960s. Based on extensive, careful observation and research on counselling sessions, Carl Rogers published *Client-centered therapy* in 1951, followed by his famous 'necessary and sufficient conditions' paper (1957) and *On becoming a person* in 1961, providing the main source of EFC. He saw the client as an expert on themselves and the counsellor as a facilitator of the *client's actualizing tendency* (the tendency of all living things to grow, adapt, and differentiate in order to prosper). This focus on the development of the client as a whole person led to the later rebranding from Client-Centred to *Person-Centred Therapy* (PCT), or more broadly as the person-centred approach (PCA).

During the 1960s and 1970s, however, students and colleagues of Rogers, including Gene Gendlin, David Wexler, and Laura Rice (eg, Wexler & Rice, 1974), continued to look more deeply at the client's process during therapy, along with specific ways that therapists could facilitate productive client process. This led to the Experiential Therapy branch of the broader Person-Centred Approach, including among others Gendlin's *Focusing* (1981) and Miller and Rollnick's *Motivational interviewing* (2012). At the same time, Laura Rice, one of the founders of EFC, began looking at what she called the *evocative function*, involving the client and therapist using vivid, metaphoric language and lively manner (Rice, 1974). In the early 1970s, after she moved to York University in Toronto, Rice also began to develop an understanding of clients as bringing particular kinds of therapeutic work to sessions, which she and her then-student Les Greenberg called *therapeutic tasks*, a reference to work on expert problem-solving in cognitive science (Greenberg, 1984b). They decided to take seriously the idea that clients are the experts on their experiences by studying how clients accomplish different kinds of therapeutic work in sessions, such as understanding puzzling personal reactions or internal conflicts. This was the seed from which the emotion-focused approach grew.

In parallel to these developments in the person-centred approach was the evolution within the broader humanistic psychology tradition of dramatic methods of psychotherapy and counselling from Psychodrama (Moreno & Moreno, 1959) and Gestalt therapy (Perls, 1969; Perls et al., 1951). Colourful and influential psychotherapists such as Jacob Moreno and Fritz Perls found that vivid enactments of aspects of self or important others could bring client experience to life and deepen therapeutic work, often more so than with words alone. In the early 1970s Les did Gestalt therapy training in Toronto and began studying transcripts of Fritz Perls' use of chair work as he and Rice developed *therapeutic task analysis*, a research method for describing the steps by which clients accomplish two kinds of therapeutic work in counselling: first, figuring out why they had a puzzling reaction to a specific situation, such as getting unexpectedly angry at a child for knocking over a cup; and, second, resolving internal conflicts, such as criticizing oneself for not being strong. These lines of research were later published in the first book to present key elements of EFT: *Patterns of change* (Rice & Greenberg, 1984).

In 1975 Les moved to the University of British Columbia and began working with his then-student Jeremy Safran to develop the emotion theory that underlies EFC; together, they published a series of influential articles (e.g., Greenberg & Safran, 1984) that culminated in their 1987 book *Emotion in psychotherapy*. Les also became interested in couples therapy, and worked with his then-student Sue Johnson to develop what they called *emotionally-focused therapy* for couples (Greenberg & Johnson, 1988; Johnson & Greenberg, 1985), one of the main variant forms of EFC.

The third founder of EFC, Robert Elliott, met Laura Rice and Les Greenberg in 1976. His first therapy trainer at UCLA was Jerry Goodman, from whom he learned Person-Centred Counselling. His early research was on counsellor response modes and the intentions behind them. After hearing Laura and Les present their work on therapeutic tasks at a conference in Wisconsin in 1977, he immediately began incorporating their approaches to client puzzling reactions and internal conflicts into his practice, subsequently adding and adapting Gendlin's Focusing, which easily fit into Laura and Les's task analysis framework.

In 1985, Greenberg, Rice, and Elliott began working together to develop an integrated form of psychotherapy that would incorporate different aspects of the broader humanistic tradition into a new, evidence-based approach based on the emerging emotion theory of Greenberg and Safran. At first they called this approach to counselling *experiential*, and later *process-experiential*; however, beginning with Greenberg and Paivio (1997), it was rebranded as *emotion-focused*.

Greenberg, Rice, and Elliott began by describing the principles that governed their practice with clients; these were refined into a set of six *practice principles* (to be described later in this chapter). This was followed by descriptions of a basic set of therapeutic tasks: *systematic evocative unfolding* (see Chapter 5) and *empathic affirmation* (Chapter 8) were based on person-centred practice; *two chair work* (Chapter 6) and *empty chair work* (Chapter 7) were based on psychodrama/Gestalt therapy; and *focusing* (Chapter 4) was adapted from Gendlin's (1981) and Cornell's (1996) writings. Elliott carried out the first study of an integrated individual EFC, with depressed clients, in the late 1980s (Elliott et al., 1990).

Practising Emotion-Focused Counselling: Pre-flight Checklist

Many people find EFC to be a demanding approach to learn, so some preparation is in order. We think you need six main things in order to be able to do Emotion-Focused Counselling (EFC) well. This set of core competences extends the humanistic counselling competences presented by Roth, Hill, and Pilling (2009) and implemented in the model of Person-Centred Experiential Counselling for Depression (Murphy, 2019).

(1) *Understand and draw on EFC emotion theory.* First, it is important for counsellors to have a grasp of EFC emotion theory (Greenberg, 2015; Greenberg & Paivio, 1997; Greenberg & Safran, 1987), including how emotion is fundamentally adaptive and the nature of the four basic dimensions of emotion: (a) kinds of emotions (sadness, anger, shame, etc.), (b) aspects of emotions (bodily, situational, etc.), (c) emotion response types (adaptive, secondary reactive, etc.), and (d) level of emotion regulation (shut-down, overwhelmed, working). By 'understand' we don't just mean an intellectual understanding of abstract concepts but rather a lived, experiential understanding of the breadth and depth of emotional experience in yourself and others. (We will describe EFC emotion theory in detail in Chapters 2 and 3.)

(2) *Adopt a person-centred but process-guiding relational stance.* Second, EFC uses a particular way of communicating with clients. The counsellor integrates 'being' and 'doing' with the client, and this results in a style that constantly balances and integrates *following* and *guiding*. As Rogers (1951) indicated, the counsellor *follows* the track of the client's internal experience as it evolves from moment to moment, remaining empathically attuned to and communicating back the client's immediate inner experience. At the same time, the counsellor actively facilitates the counselling process. Guiding does not mean lecturing the client, giving advice or insight or controlling,

pushing or manipulating the client, but rather simply offering the client potentially useful ways to work on what they want to work on. The counsellor is an experiential guide or coach who knows about subjective terrain and emotional processes. *Process guiding* is our preferred term for describing how the counsellor acts, as they offer the client opportunities to work towards what the client wants to accomplish. What this comes right down to, however, is that when disagreement occurs, or when the client and counsellor find themselves at cross purposes, the counsellor lets the client know that the client is the expert on their own experience, and acts on that basis, communicating their respect for the client's experience, even (especially!) when it is quite different from the counsellor's.

(3) *Develop an active, exploratory way of responding to clients, characterized by friendly curiosity.* Concretely, EFC counsellors express this relational stance through a distinctive pattern of specific counsellor in-session response modes, some of which will be quite familiar standard person-centred *empathic understanding responses*:

Bethany: Yeah, right now I'm feeling, kind of apprehensive.
Robert: Yeah, apprehensive, a bit concerned about what's going to happen here.

Of course, person-centred practice can vary widely in terms of how active the counsellor is and how much they reflect both what the client has said and what they *haven't* yet said but may be experiencing in the session:

Bethany: Where are you from?
Robert: So you'd like to know a bit about me before we start, is that right?

And EFC certainly uses a wider range of responding than might be found in a purely nondirective approach. For one thing, *exploratory questions* are quite important in EFC, for example:

What are you experiencing right now?

What happens inside when you hear that?

What feels important for us to look at today?

If those tears could talk, what would they say?

What has this been like for you today?

So in EFC, it's fine to ask questions; however, it's important to reflect the client's answers! At the same time, it's often more useful to offer *exploratory reflections*, which leave things more open, such as:

Bethany (hesitantly): I don't know, the feeling in my throat, it's sort of, tight?
Robert: Maybe, almost, tight? That kind of gets a bit closer to it, or…?

The main thing here is to be able to engage with your clients in a way that is both friendly, non-judgemental and at-ease, and also genuinely curious about what it is like to be them, especially feelings that are at the edge of their awareness, that are just beginning to emerge.

(4) *Learn to pick up on client markers in order to offer clients opportunities for productive therapeutic work.* EFC is marker guided. Over the years, EFC has identified a range of key indicators of different client in-session emotion-based *problem states*. These markers tell the counsellor that the client wants to work on the problem state and is ready to do so, that is, that they have an immediate, within-session goal that they want to work on. In EFC this within-session goal and the therapeutic work that goes with it are referred to as a task, a term that comes from research on expert problem solving (Greenberg, 1984b; only in this case, the client is the expert!). Counselling is therefore guided by both *perceptual skills*, which help to identify different types of emotion and problem markers, and *task skills*, which counsellors use to help the client make use of the opportunity. The work of counselling therefore involves suggesting therapeutic *experiments* that essentially involve the counsellor offering 'try this', followed by 'What do you experience?'.

EFC counsellors and researchers have studied each of the tasks in depth and over time, in order to tell us as clearly as possible what resolution looks like and how clients can get there (see Chapter 4, and Table 5.1, for the current list of EFC tasks). However, when you learn an EFC task, you can't learn it all at once; instead, you have to learn it a bit at a time, usually in the following order:

- First, you start by teaching yourself to recognize key markers (such as self-criticism).
- Second, you learn what you generally do to help clients to work with the task (such as offering two chair work).
- Third, after this, you learn the main change point in the task (such as when the critical part softens into self-compassion or regret), where the client begins moving towards resolution. (This is important so that you don't interfere with the client's process.)
- Fourth, in your work with clients over time (with the help of an EFC supervisor) you gradually teach yourself the details of how clients move from problem marker to resolution (such as learning what to do when the criticized part agrees with the critic).

This all requires patience, persistence, and a willingness to learn from and with your clients.

(5) *Realise that the counselling is not about you; instead, focus on the client's personal agency.* Counsellors, especially beginning counsellors, tend to be caught up in their own experience, especially their insecurities about their competence, their practice, and what they should be doing. Naturally, they are most aware of their own personal agency in the session, what they are supposed to do and say. We understand that, but are saying instead that the critical thing is to orient to your *clients'* personal agency, to see them as the active change agent in their counselling. Fundamentally, the counsellor in EFC tries to follow the client's experience because they recognize that the

client is a person in the same way that they are: another authentic human being who is acting in their life the best they know how, another active agent trying to make meaning, to accomplish goals, and to reach out to others. The counsellor prizes the client's initiative and attempts to help the client to make sense of their situation or resolve problems. The counsellor does this by orienting to why the client has come to counselling in general and what concerns or difficulties they have brought to work on in today's session:

Robert:	So what feels like it needs our attention today?
Bethany:	I was wondering that while I was coming here today, thinking that you were going to ask me that, but I don't know what would be best.
Robert:	Oh, so you're not quite sure what you want to work on today.
Bethany (getting a bit nervous):	Yeah, I'm not sure what would be good to do.
Robert:	Well, maybe we can take a couple minutes to help you find what would be most useful for you today.

In this situation, rather than propose something for the client to work on, the counsellor realizes that the client's initial task is to find a productive focus for the session, so they offer her the Clearing a Space task, which addresses that. (See Chapter 4 for more on Clearing a Space.)

(6) *Build up your personal resilience and courage for touching into and staying with your own and others' intense and painful emotions.* Finally, in order to do EFC, it is essential that you are able to tolerate and even dive into strong or painful emotions: not just worry, irritation, nostalgia or mild embarrassment, but terror, rage, and the deepest grieving and shame. EFC embraces the whole range of human emotions, from the most intense to the most subtle, from the most elevating to the ugliest. You may have particular emotions that you are on friendly terms with, that are easy for you to empathize with in your clients; however, you are also very likely to have other emotions that you find distasteful, objectionable or even scary. EFC asks you to develop the ability to tolerate and even to welcome the most difficult, painful emotions in yourself and others, to hold these emotions with empathy and compassion, while at the same time not getting lost in them. Developing this sort of emotional grit will probably take personal work to build your emotional resilience and courage, and is an important aspect of EFC supervision.

Emotion-Focused Counselling Practice Principles

As noted earlier, Greenberg, Rice, and Elliott began the process of developing EFC by laying out a set of six principles that guide the counsellor's relational stance and actions (Elliott, Watson, Goldman, & Greenberg, 2004; Greenberg, Rice, & Elliott, 1993; see Table 1.1).

TABLE 1.1 *Practice principles for emotion-focused counselling*

A. Relationship Principles: Facilitate Safe, Productive Therapy Relationship

---

1. *Empathic Attunement*: Enter, attend to and track the client's immediate and evolving experiencing. (Always start with this and always go back to it.)

2. *Therapeutic Bond*: Offer an empathic, caring presence to client (emotional bond aspect of alliance).

3. *Active Task Collaboration*: Offer and facilitate involvement in therapeutic work (goals and tasks).

B. Task Principles: Facilitate Work on Specific Therapeutic Tasks

---

4. *Therapist Responsiveness*: Attend carefully and differentially to important client processes (tasks, steps within tasks, client micro-processes and emotion processing modes).

5. *Emotion Transformation through Deepening*: Help clients use key therapeutic tasks to move themselves from problematic to adaptive emotions through an emotional deepening process.

6. *Client Personal Agency & Growth*: Help clients develop new emotional meaning and a sense of personal power and forward movement in their lives.

Everything in EFC is ultimately derived from these principles. The first three principles define the kind of relationship counsellors try to have with their clients and ultimately take priority over the other three principles, which describe how counsellors guide the process of therapy in order to help clients to resolve their emotional difficulties.

Relationship Principles

EFC is built on a genuinely prizing empathic relation and on the therapist being fully present, highly respectful, and sensitively responsive to the client's experience. The relationship principles involve facilitation of shared collaboration in a safe, task–focused therapeutic relationship, a relationship that is secure and focused enough to encourage the client to express and explore their key personal difficulties and emotional pain.

1. *Empathic attunement*: The counsellor enters, attends to, and tracks the client's immediate and evolving experiencing. Empathy is an evidence-based therapeutic process (Elliott, Bohart, Watson, & Murphy, 2018), and the foundation of EFC. Although it might seem simple from the outside, empathy is rich and complex, involving multiple processes and tracks. From the therapist's point of view, empathic attunement grows out of the therapist's presence and basic curiosity about the client's experiencing. It requires a series of internal actions by the therapist (cf. Greenberg & Elliott, 1997), including letting go of previously-formed ideas about the client, actively entering the

client's world, resonating with the client's experience, and feeling for and grasping the most crucial or poignant feelings or meanings at a particular moment. The counsellor always starts from empathic attunement and always comes back to it. (We will come back to empathic attunement in Chapter 4.)

2. *Therapeutic bond*: The counsellor tries to communicate empathy, caring, and presence to the client. In EFC, the client–counsellor relationship is seen as key to the change process, both directly and through providing a basis for productive therapeutic work. Thus, the counsellor seeks to develop a strong emotional bond with the client, including the three intertwined relational elements originally described by Rogers (1957): understanding/empathy, acceptance/prizing, and presence/genuineness. These conditions are expressed in many ways, both verbal and nonverbal, but in EFC we see them fundamentally as emotional states that mix curiosity, love, and compassion. In addition to understanding/empathy, acceptance is the general attitude of consistent, genuine, noncritical interest and tolerance for all aspects of the client, while prizing goes beyond acceptance to the immediate, active sense of caring for, affirming, and appreciating the client as a fellow human being, especially at moments of vulnerability. The therapist's genuine presence (Geller & Greenberg, 2012) to the client is also essential, and includes being in emotional contact with the client, being authentic (congruent, whole with self), and being appropriately transparent or open in the relationship (Lietaer, 1993), as illustrated by the example at the beginning of this chapter ('I've been doing counselling for a while, but that doesn't stop me from being a bit nervous when I start with a new person').

3. *Task collaboration*: In EFC, an effective counselling relationship also requires active partnership by both client and counsellor in both the overall goals of counselling and immediate within-session therapeutic work. Thus, in the first few sessions of EFC, the counsellor works to understand the client's view of their main presenting difficulties and to clarify the client's main, general goals for counselling. In general, the counsellor accepts the client's broad goals for counselling and their specific within-session tasks, working actively with the client to help them explore the emotional processes that drive them. In addition, the counsellor offers the client information about emotion and the counselling process, to help the client to develop a general understanding of the importance of working with emotions, and to provide rationales for specific therapeutic activities, such as two chair work. For example, towards the end of session 1, Robert offers a key piece of *experiential teaching* about the issue of the core sense of defectiveness that is so common in clients who present with social anxiety:

> *T:* I know in social anxiety there's always a sense that there's something broken in me, and that's why I'm afraid of other people, because I'm afraid they're going to see what's broken in me, so I hide, withdraw. (C: Mhm) But everybody symbolizes it in their own way. (C: OK) The thing I'm most ashamed of. Do you have words for that? (Pause) It's hard to symbolize. Do you know what I'm talking about? (C: Yeah)

Task Principles

The relationship principles are matched by three principles that guide the pursuit of therapeutic work presented by clients. These principles are expressed in the therapist's attempts to help the client to resolve internal, emotion-related problems through work on personal goals and within-session tasks. These principles have evolved a bit over the years but their essence has remained the same.

4. *Therapist Responsiveness*: Counsellors in EFC attend closely and responsively to different important client processes. These client processes include markers for starting therapeutic tasks (e.g., therapeutic alliance difficulties, unclear feelings, puzzling personal reactions to situations, unresolved relationships; see Chapter 5 for overview), steps within tasks (entry, deepening, shift points, resolution; Chapters 5–8), emotional processing modes (e.g., external story-telling, turning attention inward; Chapters 2 and 3), emotional productivity/regulation levels (dysregulated, restricted, working or change; Chapter 3), and other micro-markers such as emotional poignancy or vulnerability (Elliott et al., 2004).

5. *Emotion Transformation*: In EFC, counsellors help their clients use therapeutic tasks to move themselves from problematic to adaptive emotions through an emotional deepening process. The main tasks in EFC are not generally completed in one session. Thus, it is essential for counsellors to help clients identify the central sources of emotional pain in their lives and then to help them to work on these over several sessions. Given a choice of what to reflect, counsellors emphasize experiences associated with these main sources of emotional pain, gently persisting in offering clients opportunities to stay with these key counselling tasks. In doing so, therapists are partly guided by their knowledge of the natural emotional deepening sequence through which clients commonly move, including secondary emotions about other emotions, such as reactive anger about shame or anxiety about getting overwhelmed or feeling guilty; or core maladaptive emotions, that is, the stuck feelings that hurt the most (see Chapter 3 for more detail).

   In EFC, counsellors are guided by their knowledge of the emotional deepening sequence, as well as the specific steps within each therapeutic task. However, these are nothing like rigid recipes to be followed closely but instead are more like rough outlines for tracking client progress and offering clients opportunities for moving forward – or at least for staying out of clients' way. (We will look in depth at two of these tasks in Chapters 6 and 7).

6. *Client self-development*: Counsellors in EFC try consistently to foster client growth, empowerment, and choice. Counsellors emphasize the importance of clients' freedom to choose their actions, in counselling as well as outside it. Beyond their general stance of treating clients as experts on themselves, counsellors support their clients' potential and motivation for self-determination, mature interdependence with others, mastery, and self-development, including the development of personal power (Timulak & Elliott, 2003). Client growth is largely facilitated

through listening for and helping the client to explore the growth possibilities in their experience. For example, the counsellor might hear and reflect the assertive anger implicit in a particular client's depressed mood. Choice is facilitated in different ways, such as when the counsellor offers the client alternatives about therapeutic goals, tasks, and activities. Thus, in a particular session the counsellor might offer a hesitant client the option not to go immediately into exploration of a painful issue. We have found that clients are more willing to take risks in therapy when they feel they have the freedom to make counselling as safe as they need it to be.

Common Concerns Raised about Emotion-Focused Counselling

Before we proceed further into our description of EFC theory and practice, we feel it is important to speak to some common concerns that are expressed about EFC. These come in particular from counsellors and therapists who might describe themselves as 'nondirective' or 'classical' person-centred counsellors (e.g., Grant, 1990; Sommerbeck, 2012). We are in fact sympathetic towards these concerns, because from our point of view these represent both blocks for people learning more about EFC and also potential pitfalls for EFC practice. Thus, we take up three of the most important of these concerns here. (If you are already sold on an active, process-guiding counsellor stance based on careful distinctions between different kinds of client process, then you could skip the rest of this section, but you'll be missing some of the fun.)

Directiveness: If counsellors guide clients' processes, doesn't that turn them into powerful experts and lead to disempowering their clients? This is an old debate between EFC and the nondirective tribe of the person-centred approach (Brodley, 1990), so we want to address it up front. We have emphasized that in EFC we regard the client as the expert on their own experience, but that counsellors know a lot about different ways of working in sessions that may be useful to clients. In EFC, counsellors exercise this process expertise by offering clients things like two chair work for internal conflicts or Focusing questions about their experience of beginning therapy (as in the example at the beginning of this chapter). In the past, this process guiding has led some nondirective counsellors (e.g., Brodley, 1990) to complain that EFC counsellors are misusing their power and setting themselves up as powerful experts with their clients. Process guiding is still directiveness, they say, and therefore compromises clients' personal agency and violates unconditional positive regard.

Our response to this concern is as follows: *everything* that the counsellor does influences what the client does next (e.g., Sachse, 1990); therefore, it's impossible *not* to guide the process. The question is, how and when do we use that power? We have seen nondirective counsellors subtly discourage anxious, lost clients from asking for suggestions about what to do about their situation, by remaining silent in the face of the client's entreaty; a powerful interpersonal move indeed! Instead, EFC counsellors hold their process expertise lightly and collaboratively, offering their clients opportunities such as slowing down and looking inside (Focusing) or dialoguing with their internal critic (two chair work).

If the client for whatever reason does not want to take up the opportunity, the counsellor happily accepts this, seeing this as the client's exercise of their personal agency, their power to say no. Of course, the counsellor may be curious about the client's experience of declining the offer and is likely instead to help the client to explore their concerns or ambivalence. However, the counsellor does not try to persuade the client.

Activity Level: Do counsellors in EFC talk too much? Another frequent complaint about EFC is that it is too active, with counsellors empathically tracking clients very closely, sometimes even speaking at the same time as the client, or speaking as if they were the client (*first-person reflection*). As we said earlier, in EFC counsellors are genuinely curious and actively engaged with their clients' moment-to-moment experiencing. Here is an example of two chair work from one of Les' published videos (which also illustrates the previous point about process guiding) (Greenberg, 2007):

Les:	What are you saying [to the other part of you]?
Marcy:	Just come behind me. I'm gonna, (< .5 sec pause)
Les:	Come behind me. (0 sec)
Marcy:	Come behind me. (Les: Yeah, yeah) I'm gonna protect you. He [her husband] is not gonna hurt you no more. You're the one that keeps allowing him to, erm, do these things to you. (Les: Yes) You can stop it. Just let it go. Let it go. Let him go. (<.5 sec)
Les:	Yes. Let him go. (<.5 sec)
Marcy:	Or anybody who's hurting you, just let them go. (<.5 sec)
Les:	Right, and just come★ behind me.
Marcy:	(★Interrupting:) Just come behind me and I'll protect you. (<.5 sec)
Les:	Right. Right. Right. (Marcy: You know) So I'll keep★ him out.
Marcy:	(★Interrupting:) We don't need (voice softens:) anybody. (<.5 sec)
Les:	(Gently:) Tell her this again. (<.5 sec)
Marcy:	We don't need anybody, (Les: Yeah) just us. (.5 sec)
Les:	Just us. (.5 sec)
Marcy:	Just me and (laughs nervously) you. (<.5 sec)
Les:	Just me and you.★ Alright.
Marcy:	Yes, because I wanna be alone. When I don't wanna be with him and I'm (Les: Yeah) going through everything, I just say I wanna be alone. (Les: Right) Sometimes I want my children, I'll let my children in, sometimes I won't. (.5 sec)
Les:	Yeah, yeah. So just come behind me. (Marcy: Right) I'll keep you safe and I'll keep them out. (1 sec)
Marcy (softly:):	Right. (.5 sec)
Les:	Right, And you can just be, you and me. (.5 sec)
Marcy:	Right.

This segment is a good demonstration of the level and kind of counsellor activity in EFC. What was your response to listening to this segment in your mind's ear as you read it? Some counsellors, especially those who are used to a more nondirective or laid-back manner of relating to clients, perceive this active style of relating as intrusive or even annoying.

However, let's take a closer look at what Les and Marcy are doing in this segment. First, Les does not allow any long speeches from Marcy without offering some kind of verbal response, mostly commonly 'yeah' or 'right' (*empathic following responses*), offering roughly one word for every two words of hers. (Try counting them!) Second, he repeats, often word-for-word, each new piece of Marcy's experience as it emerges (*empathic repetition*). Third, there is no silence, and he leaves very little space between Marcy's responses and his, only slowing down when emotion begins to show itself in Marcy's voice towards the end of the segment. Overall, you can see that he is not waiting for her experience to be fully formed, or for her to finish what she has to say. Instead, he and Marcy communicate as if they are two friends who know each other well, but haven't seen each other for a while and are eager to reconnect. He thus brings quite a bit of energy to the interaction, actively constructing a shared understanding of her experience as it emerges, intensifies, and becomes more sharply (and painfully) defined.

Even if you didn't have a strong reaction to the segment, you might still be wondering how you could be so active without interrupting or becoming overbearing. However, it's not the case here that Les sets out to be as active as he is; instead, he starts by being really curious about Marcy's experience. He expects her to have interesting, unique experiences that sometimes resonate with his experiences but at other times surprise him. He wants to have an enjoyable time getting to know her and for the two of them to genuinely encounter one another as together they touch what is most poignant, special or important to her. In short, he is active because he is excited to be working with her, to experience her engaging in the work to an equal extent. It is not because he finds Marcy more interesting than other clients, but rather that he assumes that she is just as interesting in her own right as he is, or anybody else is. It's all in the attitude!

Process differentiation: How can I keep track of all the distinctions EFC makes between kinds of emotion and different processes without going into my head and losing empathy for my client's experience? Robert once made the mistake of telling one of his nondirective colleagues that he thought that there were at least eight kinds of counsellor empathy. (See Chapter 4 for more on types of empathy response.) She replied, with some confusion and even a bit of distress, 'For me, there is only one kind of empathy!' The fact is that EFC is both simple and complex. It is all about connecting empathically with our clients' deepening emotions. We always start with this and always come back to it. By the same token, this empathy leads us into deeply intricate and constantly shifting aspects of our clients' experiences, which we work to help our clients to symbolize in language as useful distinctions. What kind of anger is it, or sadness? With what kinds of inner critical voice do we mistreat ourselves, and for what reasons? EFC makes demands of both our heart and our head. Our hearts hold the empathy, follow the pain to what is most important, but then we need our heads, our reflective capacities, to work together with the client to make meaning of the experience, to collaboratively construct a guiding story with the client. That means that we don't start with the conceptual tools and try to use them to understand our clients' experiences; that is the wrong way round! Instead, we start with the feeling, and then find the sense that the feeling makes about our and our clients' lives.

Here is another way to say this: when you go into the counselling room, leave this book outside, both metaphorically and literally. After the client leaves, that's the best time for you to pick up this book, and use the distinctions to help differentiate or make sense of what happened. If we find ourselves going into our heads during the session and losing empathy for the client, that is usually because of our inner critic or coach getting in our way. (For example, 'What are you waiting for?! You should know how to do chair work by now!') These inner voices generally make us anxious, and when we get anxious, we go into our heads and forget to be empathic. It's useful to take this distraction as a sign for us to gently put the book (and our supervisor as well) aside and to refocus on the client's immediate experience, often simply by asking them where they are right now in the session. EFC's large number of concepts and terms are not programming tools; they are aids to reflection after the fact.

The Evidence on the Effectiveness of the Approach

For the past 30 years we have been collecting research on the outcomes of humanistic-experiential psychotherapies (HEPs). EFC has featured prominently in this, especially in the treatment of depression and interpersonal difficulties, including complex trauma. There are two major compilations of EFC outcome studies. The first of these (Elliott et al., 2013; see also Elliott & Greenberg, 2016) covered 1990 to 2008 and summarized the results of 34 studies of EFC, including data from more than 1,000 clients seen in either individual and couples forms of EFC. More recently, Elliott, Sharbanee, Timulak, and Watson (2019; see also Elliott et al., in press) reviewed 18 additional studies published between 2009 and 2018 and involving over 450 clients. Relational conflict and distress remain a major focus, but there is also recent work on EFC for eating difficulties and coping with chronic medical conditions.

These two meta-analyses (analyses of analyses) looked at three lines of evidence in support of EFC, which we summarize here.

The first line of evidence involved studying how much clients in EFC changed over the course of their counselling, comparing their scores on quantitative measures like the CORE Outcome Measure (Barkham et al., 2001) at the beginning of counselling to those at the end of counselling. Clients in EFC showed very large amounts of pre-post change, with even larger effects in the more recent studies. These changes were maintained at least over the course of the first year after counselling.

The second line of evidence compared clients seen in EFC of comparable people who either got no counselling or psychotherapy or were put on a waiting-list. More that 400 clients were seen in EFC in 18 controlled studies reviewed in the two meta-analyses; clients again showed very large effects when compared to would-be clients seen in no-treatment control groups. Controlled studies like these make it possible for us to conclude that there is a causal relationship between EFC and client change. More accurately, as we prefer to say, this means that clients in EFC use their counselling to cause themselves to change!

The third line of evidence compared clients in EFC to other clients seen in other kinds of non-humanistic therapy (for example, psycho-education or CBT). These comparative studies begin to help us to answer the question of whether EFC is more or less effective than other approaches outside the humanistic therapy tradition. There were 14 of these studies, comparing results from about 250 clients seen in EFC to clients seen in various forms of non-humanistic therapy. Across both meta-analyses, EFC clients did substantially better than clients seen in the non-humanistic approaches. However, a limitation of these comparative outcome studies is that they were all carried out by advocates of EFC; they are therefore vulnerable to a researcher allegiance effect, the most common form of bias in counselling outcome research. In other words, the theoretical orientation of the researcher, whether EFC or CBT, strongly affects the results, with researchers typically finding and reporting results that support their favoured approach.

In general, the existing outcome evidence for EFC most strongly supports its use with current relational distress/unresolved relational injuries. There is also strong support for its use with depression, anxiety (social and generalized), eating difficulties, and coping with chronic medical conditions.

Specifically, manualized forms of EFC have been shown to be effective in both individual and couples modalities in several randomized clinical trials (Elliott et al., 2013; Johnson, Hunsley, Greenberg, & Schlindler, 1999). A manualized form of EFC for depression, in which a number of marker guided process-guiding interventions were used within the context of an empathic relationship, has been found to be highly effective in treating depression in three separate studies (Goldman, Greenberg, & Angus, 2006; Greenberg & Watson, 1998; Watson, Gordon, Stermac, Kalogerakos, & Steckley, 2003). For example, Watson et al. (2003) found EFC to be at least as effective as Cognitive Behavioural treatment (CBT), while Goldman et al. (2006) found EFC to be more effective than person-centred counselling (PCC). Some interesting particular findings from these studies include: EFC appeared to be more effective in reducing interpersonal difficulties than either PCC or CBT; EFC also promoted more change in symptoms than PCC and was highly effective in preventing relapse (77% non-relapse; Ellison, Greenberg, Goldman, & Angus, 2009).

In Chapter 10 we come back to research on EFC and will provide a brief summary of process research on this approach.

Suggestions for Helping with the Process of Learning

We conclude this chapter with a few suggestions to facilitate your learning process. First, reading this book is only a starting point. You can't learn counselling out of a book! Please be patient with yourself. As with any complex skill, it takes a variety of learning experiences over several years to develop mastery, during which time you are likely to feel deskilled and/or self-conscious. On the other hand, reading a book can be an easily-accessible entry point. We will try throughout this book to bring EFC to life as much as we can and to make it as clear as possible.

Second, learning EFC is most effective when it combines different ways of learning: reading books like this one; watching EFC videos (see the list at the end of this chapter) or live demonstrations of more experienced EFC counsellors practising; skill practice in a safe environment, especially in the client role; real-world practice with your clients; personal supervision, especially going over your video- or audio-recordings of your practice; and personal growth work and self-reflection on what you are learning and where your blocks are.

Third, rather than expecting yourself to master EFC all at once, it will be less stressful to begin by focusing on simple, holistic understandings of tasks and treatment principles and then allowing yourself to develop progressively more complex, differentiated understandings.

Fourth, you will learn more and more quickly if you focus on trying things out rather than avoiding failure. If you put most of your attention on not making mistakes you will hold yourself back and get in your own way. Paradoxically, our advice is for you to fail faster! By this we mean, try something like two chair work, then see how your client reacts. This will work once you learn how to learn from your clients (or in skill practice, other people who are currently in the client role).

Fifth, if you have training in some other counselling approach, such as psychodynamic or CBT, don't try at first to suppress your natural way of responding. That is most likely to result in you feeling paralyzed and avoiding trying things. Your learning will proceed more smoothly if you allow yourself to work from your base of natural responding, gradually adapting what you know from those therapies into your work in EFC. If (when!) you do find yourself interpreting or problem-solving for your clients, first pay attention to exactly how your client responds to your content directive interventions (hint: clients almost never accept these interventions, although they may give token agreement out of politeness). After that, pay attention to the part of you that is pushing you to be content directive and what it is worried about.

Sixth, we believe that it is important that counsellors not force themselves into therapeutic moulds that do not suit them. We are very aware that EFC appeals strongly to some, but not all, counsellors, just as it appeals strongly to many, but not all, clients. Although research is lacking, EFC probably works best with clients seeking an active, intense counselling experience, who are not completely cut off from their emotions, and who don't need their counsellor to be a content expert. EFC should not be imposed on clients who find that it clashes with their values and perceived needs. In the same way, it should not be imposed on counsellors whose skills, preferences or world-view run in other directions than those best suited to EFC, for example, counsellors who feel a strong need to exercise their expertise, or who simply find other approaches more appealing. Although we have our own values and preferences, we are firm believers in theoretical and clinical pluralism, of 'letting a thousand flowers bloom'.

Finally, remember that, in the end, your clients are your best teachers of this or any form of counselling, once you learn how to listen for what they are telling you. That's why empathic attunement is the core of EFC practice. If you start by entering your clients' moment-by-moment experiencing, you will be able to see and hear how they take what you offer them, and you will be able to learn from that, and keep on learning. The two of us have each been doing therapy for nearly 50 years, and we continue to learn from each new client. That's the adventure of EFC!

Introducing Our Two Case Examples

In this book we will feature two clients as running examples of EFC, using their counselling to illustrate concretely what EFC looks like and how it unfolds over time. Each of these clients has had various details, including their names, altered to protect their identity.

Bethany. You have already met Bethany, whose entrance into counselling opened this chapter. She was a 33-year old Scottish woman, married and with a two-year-old daughter. She came to counselling to get help with her fear of other people ('social anxiety'), which was interfering with her relationships with others, both in social situations and in close personal relationships. As part of a research project, before starting counselling she met with a researcher, who, among other things, helped her to construct an individualized outcome measure called the Personal Questionnaire. On this instrument, Bethany listed nine problems that she wanted to work on during her counselling. This list, which she ranked in order of importance, gives a pretty good idea of her presenting issues and concerns:

1.   I get anxious.
2.   I find meeting new people very stressful.
3.   I worry a lot about what people think of me.
4.   I am scared of embarrassing myself by doing something wrong.
5.   I get overwhelmed by my anxiety.
6.   I find it hard to trust and open up to friends.
7.   I find it stressful having people to my home.
8.   I get overly defensive quite quickly.
9.   I notice that I punish myself or am hard on myself (too much).

Bethany was seen by Robert, a 65-year-old European-American clinical psychologist who was living in Scotland, for 19 sessions of EFC.

Jonah. Jonah was a 40-year-old European Canadian man who completed 16 sessions of therapy. He was married, had one son and came to counselling reporting that he wanted to get rid of his depression, which he attributed to a recently suffered financial loss. He was afraid he was getting worse and that his depression was interfering with his work and his relationships. He said he had a tendency to not let anybody in, and that he dealt with depression by going to sleep. He was seen by a 46-year-old European Canadian female psychologist, whom we will call Margaret and who was supervised by Les.

Further Exploration

Reading

Elliott, R. (2012). Emotion-focused therapy. In P. Sanders (Ed.), *The tribes of the person-centred nation: An introduction to the schools of therapy related to the person-centred approach* (2nd ed., pp. 103–130). Ross-on-Wye, UK: PCCS Books.

Watching

Elliott, R., (2016). *How Robert Elliott came to Emotion-focused Therapy.* Counselling Channel. Available at: www.youtube.com/watch?v=uTJh8PQKNco

Greenberg, L. S. (2016). *Interview Juliette Becking and Les Greenberg about EFT.* APANTA/Eduseries. Available at: https://vimeo.com/157982795/2a8c8b3251

Reflecting

1. What initially drew your attention to the emotion-focused approach? What do you think having read this chapter?
2. What do you think about the common concerns we discussed earlier in this chapter? Which ones do you share?
3. What is your response to strong emotions, such as rage, panic or deep grief, in yourself or other people? How might this affect you in working with clients?

2

Emotion Theory in Emotion-Focused Counselling

Definition and Importance of Emotion

Before we explore in more detail how to counsel clients in an emotion-focused way, it's important for us to tell you about what emotions are and how they work. Learning the basic theory on which EFC is based can be challenging, so we will try to present it in as clear a manner as possible, using figures, boxes, and tables, and illustrating the concepts with material from our running cases.

Emotion is the feeling of what is happening (Damasio, 1999). Emotion is an emergent property that is greater than the sum of its parts and provides the quality, intensity, and meaning of our experiences. In brief, we can define emotion as an emergent, holistic process that...

- points to what is important to us in the situations of our lives,
- prepares us to take useful actions in those situations,
- is experienced in our bodies,
- is usefully represented with words or images, and
- organizes self/tells us who we are.

We may consciously and directly experience our emotions ourselves, or we may observe them operating implicitly in others.

Emotions and organismic valuing. Rogers (1959) referred to a fundamental *organismic valuing process* at the centre of the actualizing tendency. Similarly, Perls (1969) referred to a process of actualizing the self and to the wisdom of the organism. He saw these as guiding us to become who we really are rather than trying to get us to become what we are not. However, from the perspective of EFC, Rogers and Perls did not spell out the basic processes of organismic valuing/wisdom and actualizing as fully as they could have. Furthermore, these approaches used a narrow definition of emotion and downgraded it as secondary to the actualizing tendency and the organismic valuing process.

In EFC, emotion is the fundamental concept of human experience, overlapping to some extent with Rogers' organismic valuing process. Emotions are defined by most emotion theorists as arising from automatic evaluations of situations in relation to needs (Ekman & Davidson, 1994; Frijda, 1986). Emotion is the moment-by-moment feeling of what is good for us or bad for us and acts as our most fundamental guide (Zajonc, 1980). In short, emotions tell us if things are going our way and prepare us to deal effectively with situations. This description closely parallels the concept of the organismic valuing process.

EFC holds that the organismic valuing process can be deconstructed as emotion in action and sees emotion as fuelling the self-actualizing process. Thus, from an EFC perspective, our emotions are the basis of Rogers' and Perls' organismic wisdom, providing the foundation for who we most fundamentally are. We argue in this chapter that different kinds of emotions, like fear, anger, sadness, etc., are different kinds of bodily wisdom about what is happening for us, if we simply listen carefully. Emotion can even be as subtle as feeling that something you tell yourself isn't right. For example, early in session 2 of Bethany's counselling, her counsellor is having her make a list of and set aside all the things that are keeping her from feeling good. After she has identified and cleared away four of her current sources of distress, she says:

Bethany: [a little hesitantly:] I… think that's everything.

Robert: So say to yourself, to check, 'If it wasn't for those four things, let's see, there's the mother-in-law, the wasting time, the worrying about getting upset about little things, and my visit to my parents. If it wasn't for those things, I'd feel great.' (Bethany laughs) Try saying that to yourself and see what happens.

Bethany: If it wasn't for all those things, I, would, feel great.

Robert: And what happens when you say that?

Bethany: I don't really believe it.

Robert: You don't believe it, there's something else! (laughing) Right, OK. So what else is there? (small pause) What else would keep me from feeling great? (pause)

Bethany: I think just in general not being happy about myself.

So here, in this little example, we see the bodily wisdom of emotion in action in several ways: first, in identifying four things that are bothering her; second, in being able to easily check whether a description of an emotional state ('feeling fine') fits her experience or not, and finally, what the previously unnoticed distress was about.

In fact, we are arguing here that each of the different kinds of emotions is its own special kind of wisdom. Fear, for example, is the wisdom of recognizing and coping with danger by avoiding it or making preparations to reduce it. Anger is the wisdom of recognizing when our boundaries are being violated and taking steps to maintain those boundaries. (Of course, as we will elaborate, not all fear or anger is wise; the point is to know which is which.)

The importance of emotions. Emotion, at its core, is an adaptive system that has evolved to help us survive and thrive. Emotions are connected to our most essential needs. Emotions rapidly alert us to situations important to our well-being and tell us if things are going our way or not (Greenberg, 2010). To elaborate the fear example from the previous paragraph, our emotion system tells us when we are in danger, it sets fear processing in motion, guiding our attention to search for cues of danger and readying us to take adaptive action, action towards meeting our needs for safety. Emotion also leads to thought ('cognition') and so we then begin to be consciously aware of thinking fearful thoughts.

At their best, emotions are healthy and help us survive and thrive. They give meaning to life and intensity to relationships. They orient us adaptively to the environment, and help us create meaningful bonds with others. They help us to escape danger, to stand up for what's right, seek comfort when needed, and to help others in need. At their worst, they become maladaptive: they make us feel not good enough; lead us to withdraw from others; bring on panic about things that aren't likely to happen; or raise feelings about being abandoned or alone in the world. They also can result in destructive behaviour, such as becoming overly submissive or people-pleasing, or engaging in risky or destructive behaviour that hurts us and the ones we love.

In this chapter we summarize what we know about emotions. In particular, we present a model of human emotion as consisting of four fundamental dimensions, which define its richness and variability:

I. Emotion scheme components (e.g., situational-perceptual)
II. Emotional intensity (level of emotion regulation; e.g., overwhelmed)
III. Emotion categories (e.g., happy, sad)
IV. Emotion response types (adaptiveness; e.g., secondary reactive)

Working effectively with our clients' emotions will require that we pay attention to all four of these dimensions. In Chapter 3 we provide an up-to-date account of how EFC counsellors put all this together to help their clients transform their emotions through a stepwise process of emotional deepening.

Emotion Schemes: What are Emotions Made of?

The basis of human experience. Children come into the world with inborn programmes for a range of emotions, including sadness, anger, and fear. We don't teach them how to be angry, sad, or afraid. But what they become angry at, sad about, or afraid of is developed through experience. Emotion schemes are our internal representations of our lived experience. They are based on inborn emotional responses coupled with lived experience of that emotion; together these form more complex internal organizations which also, with development, come to include thoughts and beliefs. For example, you may have an emotion scheme based on shame that incorporates a set of lived experiences, including disapproval from your mother, being teased as a child, experiences of failure at football, not being popular at school, and being humiliated by a teacher, coupled with beliefs formed from shameful experiences and internalization of criticisms. These emotion-based schemes, when activated by criticism at your work, rapidly and automatically produce felt experience and action tendencies and form the foundation of a self who feels worthless and often reacts with shame.

Damasio (1999), a leading neuroscientist, in his book titled *The feeling of what happens* suggested that human consciousness first emerged in the form of unverbalized feelings, before we developed language. Damasio argued that awareness comes into being in the story of the effects that external objects have on our body states. Knowing first arises as a feeling of what happens to our body. So for example, the toy that I trip over leads me to fall down and hurt myself, or my mother's breast feeds me milk and it feels good. Essentially, in making sense of these experiences, we inferred 'This happened to me when that occurred and affected my body state in this way'. This experience forms the basis for an emotion scheme. These experiences are first coded as wordless narratives that we understand long before we can speak. Then, when these schemes are articulated in language, they become our very first conscious stories that help us make sense of our life experiences. In this way, our ancestors increasingly evolved the ability to link together the effects that objects, events, and people have on their felt bodies. Eventually we developed the ability to symbolize these emotion schemes in the form of gestures and language, so that we could pass them along to others in the form of stories, stories that have beginnings, middles and ends, agents, objects and intentions, all strung together in time-ordered sequences that convey our understanding of what causes what.

EFC's expanded concept of emotion. As we said earlier, EFC expands the concept of emotion beyond what Rogers and others meant. Emotion schemes themselves are unconscious and automatic; they are therefore not directly available to awareness. However, they can be identified through the experiences they produce. Experience is available to awareness, and can be attended to, explored, and made sense of by a process of activation, attention and reflection. Paying focused attention to bodily feelings is very useful for bringing automatic emotional information into explicit, verbalizable experience that will be remembered. The way we find ourselves to be in a situation, that is, the feeling of what happens (for example, feeling put down, confident or shy) emerges from one or more emotion schemes being activated and then manifesting themselves as bodily feelings. Our implicit emotional state can then become what we consciously feel by first paying attention to it, then symbolizing it in awareness, reflecting on it, and forming narratives that explain it. In the process we create the self that we become in that moment (Greenberg & Pascual-Leone, 1995). We thus are in a continual process of simultaneously discovering and creating who we are.

Emotion schemes, especially as embedded in memories of emotion episodes, can be seen as networks of interlinked components of experience. It is useful to distinguish five broad aspects or domains within emotion schemes (see Figure 2.1):

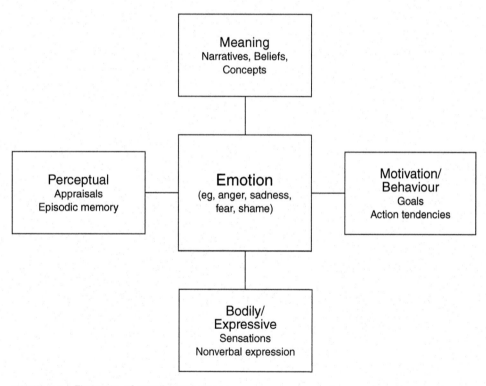

FIGURE 2.1 *Elements of emotion schemes*

- How we *perceive* the present situation and *remember* past situations,
- What we experience in our *bodies* and express through them,
- The meanings or *symbolic representations* of things (words, metaphors, identities, narratives),
- Our needs and action tendencies, and
- The implicit or experienced *feelings* themselves.

(a) The *perceptual/situational* component represents the person's past or current environments and includes immediate perceptions of the current situation. How we see things may include sensory memories or memories of specific events. Thus, a person may hear a sound or see an object that evokes a memory, or remember an emotion-laden episode like being left on the doorstep in her pretty party dress waiting for her father to pick her up when he never came. For example, when Robert's client Bethany reported in session 1 that she felt apprehension about starting counselling, he asked her:

Robert: Do you have a sense of what the apprehension's about, what it's pointing to?
Bethany: Yeah, talking to people about emotions and stuff is difficult. So it's, apprehensive about what might come up.

This is another way of saying that emotions are always *about* something; they always point to something in the person's situation, immediate or general, past or present. It is also the case that our feelings are always part of a story or narrative (Sarbin, 1989), although in some cases the story may be implicit or buried (*unstoried emotions*; Angus & Greenberg, 2011).

(b) The *bodily/expressive* component includes immediate and automatic bodily sensations such as a tight feeling in the gut accompanied by tension in shoulders, or butterflies in the stomach and constricted breathing as well as nonverbal expressions of emotion, such as a facial grimace or a reflexive pushing away gesture in the hands and arms. For example, Bethany described the bodily sensation that accompanied her apprehension about starting counselling as a tightness in her throat.

Emotion expresses itself in distinctive bodily responses to various situations that our ancestors encountered even before language was developed. Our hearts are predisposed to race when we see looming objects, snakes, crawling insects or large moving shadows at night, or when we hear loud noises or the screams of fellow humans. The racing heart and the other physiological changes that occur under these conditions collectively serve as a danger detector. They occur under these situations; some of this response is innate, while some is learned. When the emotion is activated, it produces the appropriate physiological changes. Not only do bodily processes facilitate emotions, but emotions also influence bodily processes. For example, we now recognize that what people refer to as 'stress' is an undifferentiated bodily experience of unresolved emotions like anger, fear, sadness, and shame. Emotion has also been clearly connected to the immune system and physiology (Pennebaker & Seagal, 1999).

(c) The *meaning* component will carry the semantic meaning in language, including verbal statements such as 'If it's worth doing at all, it's worth doing perfectly'; metaphorical qualities/images like 'wound up tight like a coil'; identity beliefs like 'I'm a failure' or 'I'm a victim'; or narratives like 'I ruin all my relationships and am going to end up all alone'. When Robert asked Bethany if she could come up with an image or metaphor for her apprehension, she said:

Bethany: OK. I mean I guess it kind of feels like, a bomb. You know, like the apprehension is usually a precursor to the anxiety.

In addition to the pre-verbal emotion system organized around emotion affect regulation, we have a second general system: a meaning construction system based on symbols and language. Narrative is the main way of constructing meaning and we all possess a will to create stories and meaning (Angus & Greenberg, 2011). Frankl (1946/2006) proposed there is a will to meaning and showed us how those who have a reason to live can bear with almost any situation. We are born meaning makers who construct our realities by creating the stories that in turn guide us (Bruner, 1991). It is impossible for us to not create meaning. Interaction between the pre-verbal emotion regulation and the meaning creation systems determines experience. Emotions then are what move us while the meaning we create from them is what we live by.

(d) The *need/action tendency* component includes the goal or aim of the emotion to obtain comfort, safety or protection of boundaries plus the action tendency to approach, to flee or to assert.

Robert:	And what does that apprehension make you want to do?
Bethany:	Yeah, like, leave (laughs)
Robert:	Leave! Yeah, like something is saying, 'Get the heck out of there!' (C: mhm) 'This is not safe.' (C: mhm) Where would you go? What's it telling you?
Bethany:	(shrugs shoulders) Either just leave the room, or like if my husband was here, I'd just let him (laughing) do all the talking.

Many people (including emotion theorists such as Frijda, 1986) believe that basic human needs drive emotions. (Similarly, Rogers (1959) held that the actualizing tendency drove emotions.) However, from an emotion-focused perspective, emotions generate needs, rather than the other way around; emotions, rather than needs, are the basic psychological units that provide the values or preferences that push us in one direction or another. Thus, rather than put forward a set of motivations, such as attachment, autonomy, creation of meaning or control, as basic, EFC sees that needs are constructed from basic emotional sensitivities with which we are born, emerging out of our experience of interacting with others.

(e) Finally, the *consciously experienced or implicit emotion* is the integrated sum of the different emotion scheme elements and provides the feeling of what is happening; as we have been saying, it is an emergent property that is greater than the sum of its parts and provides the quality, intensity, and meaning of the experience. In Bethany's case, the newly emerging experienced emotion of apprehension came first and then she was able to use the Focusing task (see Chapter 5) offered to her to elaborate the emotion scheme elements that made up her feeling of what was happening as she began counselling.

Thus, to sum up the role of emotion schemes, we continually interpret, transform, and derive meaning from the information that comes from our senses, both from the environment and from inside our body. We then interpret these outer and inner sensations and attach them to other sensations, forming a larger meaning. Then we find responses that are aimed at internal satisfaction, as well as harmony with the demands and expectations of the environment. The resulting activity in our brain and nervous system becomes an emotion scheme structure that, when activated, creates the flow of our experience. Feeling an emotion involves experiencing body changes in response to the evoking object or situation, informed by past emotional experiences. This is the EFC account of Rogers' (1959) organismic valuing process.

Emotional experience produced by these structures as well as providing our more basic, biologically-based emotional responses like anger, fear, and sadness also provide both higher order feelings, such as being on top of the world or down in the dumps, and our sense of things, such as a sense of danger or of attraction (Damasio, 1999; Greenberg & Safran, 1987). These emotional responses have been informed by experience and benefited from learning. Much automatic adult emotional experience is of this higher order, generated by learned, idiosyncratic emotion schemes that influence decision making by helping us to anticipate future outcomes.

An example of this second, higher level, more cognitively complex, type of emotion would be the feeling in the pit in our stomach that we might experience upon unexpectedly encountering an ex-partner. The trigger is clearly acquired, but the process is still automatic and often unverbalized. Regardless of whether or not the experience *can subsequently* be fully put into words, the tacitly generated experience nonetheless influences us. These memory-based emotion schemes guide appraisals, bias decisions, and serve as blueprints for physical arousal and action. They act as crucial guides, which we often need to refer to, and help us reason and make decisions. These perceptual/bodily/cognitive/motivational emotion schemes are thus a central focus of EFC. When emotion schemes become problematic, as we describe later in this chapter, they become important targets for therapeutic work (Greenberg & Paivio, 1997).

Integrating biology and culture. All people, regardless of when and where they are born, come into the world with the same evolutionarily adaptive emotional system that serves as the basis for our common humanity. It is true that our individual experiences, including our cultures, put an indelible stamp on our emotions, sometimes even twisting and distorting them into something we or others no longer recognize. Culture and experience train us to hide emotions or to express them in unique ways. Depending on what different families or cultures may view as natural or acceptable, they may express themselves, for example, by having a stiff upper lip, or by dancing joyously in the streets during Mardi Gras. Despite varied experience and training, however, we are all pretty much alike. Your family may believe in the importance of feelings, while my family may view feelings as weak and undesirable. Similarly, my culture may highly value self-effacing humility, while your family may prize brash assertiveness.

Because different cultures often have different rules of emotional expression, culturally sensitive counsellors need to be aware of their own and others' cultural views about different emotions and when/how they should be expressed as opposed to being suppressed or interrupted. Being a culturally sensitive counsellor involves first recognizing and understanding one's own culture and how it influences one's relationship with a client, and then understanding and responding respectfully to the culture that is different from one's own. However, beneath all the different rules about when, where, and how much to display different emotions, there lies a common core of emotional human-ness that makes it possible for us as fellow humans to understand each other regardless of culture, or, for that matter, minority status, gender, sexual orientation or disability.

Emotions and the brain. Emotions and the body are inextricably linked. In particular, we now know that the limbic system (a part of the mid-brain possessed by all mammals) is responsible for basic emotional processes, such as fear (LeDoux, 1996). The limbic system influences physical health by governing many of the body's physiological processes, including the immune system and most major body organs. LeDoux (1996) found that there are two paths for producing emotion: (a) the fast 'low' road, via which the amygdala (a key part of the limbic system) senses danger and broadcasts an emergency distress signal to the brain and the body, and (b) the slower 'high' road, whereby the same information is processed more slowly in the neocortex (the newer outer part of the brain where we think). Because the shorter amygdala pathway transmits signals more than twice as quickly as the neocortex route, we are rapidly oriented to the world and automatically prepare ourselves to take survival-oriented action. All this occurs before we think, and the thinking brain often cannot intervene in time to stop these emotional responses. Thus, the automatic emotional response occurs before we can stop it, whether it be jumping back from a snake, snapping at a spouse or crying at a funeral. In some situations, it is clearly adaptive to respond quickly, whereas at other times, better functioning results from the guiding of emotion through reflection. This involves bringing cognition to emotion and integrating reason and emotion.

Emotional Intensity and Emotion Regulation

The second dimension of emotional experience is emotional intensity. Feelings vary along a wide spectrum, from very subtle, mild or fleeting to highly charged, strong or pervasive. This range of emotions is of great value in helping us meet the wide variety of human situations. Both quiet satisfaction and intense joy have their place. Nevertheless, in general, emotions tend to be most useful when they fall into the middle or 'Goldilocks' range: neither too cool or too hot.

On the one hand, an emotion that is too mild is going to have trouble getting our attention; we will have trouble receiving the valuable information it is trying to convey to us. Similarly, we might be stopping ourselves from feeling our emotions (*over-regulating* them) by pushing them far away from us, blocking ourselves from feeling them or making ourselves numb. (In EFC, we call this self-blocking of emotions *self-interruption*.) Not being aware of emotion at all or not sensing what we feel in our body makes exploration and problem solving intellectual. There is no emotional information to orient us to the situation or to act to satisfy needs or attain our goals. In addition, lack of emotion awareness can lead to a type of bottled-up blow-up syndrome, where we suddenly go from being unexpressive to bursting into anger or sadness.

On the other hand, an emotion that is too strong is likely to overwhelm us, leaving us *under-regulated*. This can take various forms:

• Chaotic and scattered by too many worries,
• Disorganized with panic,
• Out of control with rage,

- Inconsolable with endless grief, or
- Immobilized with shame.

But when our emotions become too strong, we may not be able to hear what they are trying to tell us either: it's as if they are shouting too loud for us to hear the message. Instead of us having our emotions, it's like they are having us (Greenberg, 2002). Often, we simply shut down, just like when our house electrical system gets overloaded and throws a circuit breaker or burns out a fuse, flipping between under-regulation and over-regulation.

In these situations, we need to find ways to regulate our emotions. When they are blocked or too mild, we want to activate them to bring them up into the moderate range where we will be able to use their valuable information to help us find useful ways of responding. When they are too loud, we will want to moderate them so that we can stay in touch with them in order to hear what they have to say.

Emotion regulation is the master process in EFC: the need to manage our various emotions so that they work to our benefit and help us get our needs met. So we try to enhance pleasant emotions, like love towards a valued other, happiness about pleasant events, curiosity about new or unusual things, or pride at accomplishment. Frequently, we find ourselves trying to reduce our unpleasant feelings, such as fear of danger, sadness at loss, anger about injustice, or shame at failure. In spite of this, emotion regulation is not simply about increasing pleasant feelings and reducing distressing or unpleasant ones. After all, the function of unpleasant emotions is to draw our attention to important difficulties in our immediate situation, so that we can address them appropriately, by containing or escaping the danger, by restoring something of what was lost, by correcting the injustice, or by motivating ourselves to try harder so that next time we will succeed. When the adaptive action succeeds in coping with the difficult situation, the distressing emotion goes away, and we feel better. Emotion regulation!

We first learned to regulate our emotions from our parents or primary caregivers. Ideally, they comforted us when we were upset and got us excited when we were feeling sleepy or unmotivated. Over time, we internalized their example and began to regulate our emotions for ourselves. Unfortunately, in many cases, our caregivers over-regulated our emotions, scolding us for being over-exuberant, shaming us as 'cry-babies' or for 'whinging' when we were sad, warning us sternly if we showed signs of pride at accomplishment, and so on. As a result, we learned to over-regulate our emotions.

For example, Jonah, whom we introduced in Chapter 1, had been depressed since he was a teenager and had dealt with it mainly by sleeping. He had had a very punitive mother, who criticized him all the time; because of this he had withdrawn from conflict with her and become submissive in order to avoid discord with her; he now did the same with his wife. Thus, Jonah had learned to over-regulate most of his feelings, especially anger and sadness. As a result, he shut himself down and became resigned and depressed.

A key issue in emotion regulation is not so much a matter of how intense our emotions are but whether we feel safe with them or not. If they feel out of control, we fear where our strong feelings might take us and what that might do to us.

In these situations, we try to contain them or shut them down. We stop listening to the information they are trying to tell us and instead focus on getting rid of them. In some situations, this is necessary. However, it's easy for this to become the other form of emotion dysregulation: over-regulation. We will come back to issues of emotion regulation in Chapter 3.

Emotion Categories: What Kinds of Emotions are There?

A third emotional dimension is the kind or category of emotion. Emotion theorists love to make up lists or systems for kinds of emotions. Decades and even centuries (Gendron & Barrett, 2009) have been spent trying to come up with the best system of categories (e.g., Ekman, 1992) or dimensions (Plutchik, 1991) for classifying emotions. As far as we can tell, no definitive answer is possible to the question of how many and what kinds of emotions there are. Being practical souls, EFC counsellors are not very interested in coming up with a master list of emotions; we are more interested in simply getting on with helping people sort out their emotional difficulties. What we can say for the purposes of EFC is that there is a not-too-long list of emotions that turn out to be important in working with clients.

Our current entries for the most frequently occurring and important emotions in EFC are discussed below and summarized in Table 2.1.

TABLE 2.1 *Key emotions in EFC*

Situation	Emotion	Need: Adaptive Action
Loss of someone or something important	**Sadness**	Comfort: express hurt (alternatively: disengage)
Violation (attack on self, family, possessions, goals, values)	**Anger**	Protect boundaries or energize self: assert, strike out
Danger (Anxiety: possible danger)	**Fear/anxiety**	Safety: flee, freeze, seek protection (Anxiety: monitor, prepare)
Having acted inappropriately or revealed a social defect	**Shame**	Protect or repair social standing, connection with others: hide, correct or express awareness of impropriety
Harming a valued other	**Guilt**	Repair the damage: apologize, make amends
Offensive, dirty, indigestible object or person	**Disgust**	Reject noxious object or person: expel, avoid
Psychological injury	**Emotional pain**	Disengage to prevent further injury: withdraw into self to heal if possible

(Continued)

TABLE 2.1   *(Continued)*

Situation	Emotion	Need: Adaptive Action
Novel, unknown, unexpected stimuli	**Interest/ curiosity**	Explore, understand: attend, approach, engage, immerse
Achievement of goal, task, need or connection	**Joy/happiness**	Savour and share: stop and appreciate, let others know, strengthen connections
Suffering of a vulnerable other	**Compassion**	Provide caregiving: offer comfort, soothing, support, validation

Note: Compiled and adapted from Greenberg & Paivio (1997)

Sadness seeks comfort when there is loss. Sadness is an attachment signal: it tells us we have lost someone or something important. This could be a parent, partner, child or friend, but also includes the loss of hopes, dreams, and possibilities. Sadness can take the form of grief or sorrow, but also disappointment, despair or hopelessness. When we experience sadness, we may feel the need to cry, or to reach out in some way and communicate to others a need for comfort and support to help cope. Conversely, we may become quiet or lethargic and withdraw from others. (In EFC, we recognize these are two different kinds of sadness: connecting sadness and disengaging sadness.)

Anger asserts when there is violation. Anger is a boundary violation signal: it tells us that some kind of personal boundary is being violated, that some kind of unwanted intrusion is in progress. This can include something standing in the way of our achieving something (= violation of goals or agency); it also includes injustice (= violation of fairness or important values), telling us that we or people we care about are being treated unfairly. When angry, people often feel strong and more powerful and feel the urge to assert themselves or even strike out. Through displaying anger, people meet the need of boundary protection or energize themselves to overcome obstacles. Anger can mobilize us out of stuckness or despair.

Fear/anxiety seeks safety when there is danger. Fear/anxiety is a danger signal: it tells us that someone or something is threatening us or someone we love. It could be a dangerous person, animal, situation or disease. If the danger is immediately present, we call it fear; if the danger is possible or in the future, we call it anxiety. We often experience this emotion with shortness of breath, pounding heart and tight chest; sometimes we freeze. Specifically, *fear* motivates us to flee from what's threatening, to freeze in order to not attract attention, or to seek protection from others; while *anxiety* motivates us to take precautions to avoid or prepare ourselves for danger or catastrophe. Fear/anxiety helps us meet the need of safety. This emotion is strongly connected to feeling attached to caregivers and is activated when those bonds are threatened (= separation anxiety).

Shame seeks to protect our status/connections when we have violated social norms. Humans are social animals, and so we have evolved social emotions, including shame.

Shame is a social status damage signal: it tells us that we have behaved inappropriately or are in some way socially defective. When expressed, it tells others that we are aware of the norm violation. (Violating norms while not being aware of doing so – 'having no shame' – is a worse violation than simple norm violation.) The experience of shame is the feeling of not being worthy or good enough in the eyes of others who are important to us, such as family, friends or society in general. Shame might also be a reaction to being humiliated by others or feeling that something is really wrong with us. We typically feel shame as an urge to hide and not be seen. However, it also motivates us to try to correct or repair the impropriety or defect, and with that our damaged social status and connections to others. *Expressed shame* is part of this repair process. By showing others our shame, we communicate our desire and ability to do better; based on this, we are asking to be invited back into the group and to feel once again that we belong. The underlying need is to be accepted and acknowledged, or at least not rejected or judged negatively.

Guilt seeks to repair harm to a valued other whom we have injured or let down. A related social emotion is guilt. Guilt is a relational injury signal, telling us that we have harmed another person who is important to us in some way. Usually, the other is a person close to us, such as a parent, partner, child or ourselves; however, it can also include our work colleagues or clients, others we don't know (such as refugees or our descendants), and even abstract entities, like God, our country or the environment. The immediate need with guilt is to repair the damage we have done by apologizing and trying to make amends. The underlying need is to restore our image of ourselves as good people.

Disgust rejects what is bad for us. Disgust is a noxious stimulus signal: it tells us that we are in the presence of something noxious or bad for us that we must push away and not let into our body. When exposed to a noxious smell or object, we react automatically, moving our heads away from the smell and displaying the recognizable facial expression of disgust (Ekman & Friesen, 1969). The noxious input can be a dirty or indigestible object or substance, but can also include an offensive, abusive or harmful person. The need is to reject, avoid or expel the noxious substance or experience.

Emotional pain disengages to prevent further injury. We round out our list of distressing emotions with the most basic one. Emotional pain is a non-specific psychological injury signal: it tells us that something in us has been damaged, that we are broken inside and that this needs attention. This is a highly undifferentiated emotion. It is strong distress without a specific focus: all we know is that something feels broken inside us (Bolger, 1999). Emotional pain feels like physical pain, but there is no obvious physical injury or illness. Our stomach may hurt; it can feel like our heart is broken; sometimes we are left with a kind of ache in our body, like an old wound that has never properly healed. The need here is to withdraw into self, to disengage from the world. This is undoubtedly an ancient evolutionary response. We feel like a cat or some other wounded animal that crawls away to hide somewhere safe to conserve its resources; we just need to lay low, to keep safe while we either heal or die. Emotional pain colours other emotions, especially sadness and shame, reinforces their action tendency to disengage or withdraw, but has a distinctive emotional quality and is often what our clients first present to us in counselling.

So far we have been discussing distressing emotions. We don't call them 'negative emotions' because in EFC we see them in a positive rather than a negative light. They are valuable, even necessary, for survival, because they tell us something is wrong that needs attention. These are the emotions our clients bring to counselling. However, particularly as counselling progresses, other, more pleasurable emotions begin to emerge and provide valuable resources for clients.

Interest/curiosity explores new or unusual things. Interest/curiosity is novelty signal: it tells us that there is something in front of us that is novel, unexpected or unusual and motivates us to explore as a possible resource. We are, after all, descended from hunter-gatherers who often found themselves in marginal or unknown environments; they needed to constantly search for potential food or other resources. Interest/curiosity involves an opening up, a broadening of our attention. There is an urge to approach and explore the novel. This could be discovering something new, learning to know something, immersing ourselves in hobbies or work, or approaching other people. We experience this emotion as a kind of anticipation, excitement or focus, and this prompts us to approach: I wonder what's over there? What is that? Who is that? What could I do with that? The need is getting to explore and immerse, thus gaining resources, not just food or materials for making things, but also a partner, knowledge or self-realization.

Joy/happiness savours and shares the meeting of needs. Joy/happiness is a need satisfaction signal: it tells us that something good has happened to us or that we have achieved something important. Examples include being with good friends who acknowledge us and wish us well; finally getting through a difficult period of our life; feeling safe again after a threat; or seeing that someone we care about is doing well. This might come with a sense of well-being; we might feel tension release that we didn't even know was there or suddenly get the urge to smile or laugh. We might express this to others, letting them know that we are feeling well and enjoying their company. In this way, joy/happiness also fosters closeness and belonging, and needs to be both savoured and shared.

Compassion takes care of the vulnerable. Compassion is a caregiving signal: it tells us that a vulnerable other is suffering and needs us to take care of them. Humans give birth to young who are too vulnerable to care for themselves and therefore require extended caregiving compared to other mammals and other animals (Portmann, 1897/1990). To cope with this, they evolved a high level of compassion for small, vulnerable creatures like their newborn infants (Goetz, Keltner, & Simon-Thomas, 2010). Moreover, this compassion extends to a range of vulnerabilities in others, including emotional vulnerability such as sadness and fear. Importantly, we can even offer compassion to ourselves when we are feeling vulnerable. The need in compassion is to provide care, comfort, soothing or support for those (including ourselves) who need it.

Complexity of emotions. However, as you've been reading through our list of therapeutically important emotions, you may have noticed that they have all been relatively straightforward: situation → emotion → need/adaptive response. These are all simple emotions; they are more like basic emotional elements with a relatively simple structure. In contrast, our more difficult emotions generally feel much more muddled than that, more tangled, blended or layered. We will have more to say about emotional sequences and layers in the next section of this chapter and also in the next chapter, but for now we want to note that there are many blends or more specific varieties of emotion that have a distinct emotional flavour of their own. An EFC counsellor earns their keep by being able to understand more than the simple emotions; most often we are trying to help our clients access and put into words these more complicated or subtle emotions.

Emotion Response Types

Because emotion has historically been contrasted with reason or thinking, academics have treated emotion as a single class of events for the purposes of contrasting them with reason. All emotions, however, are not the same. First, although each emotion (e.g., anger) has a distinct form and function, it has many variations. As we have said, in anger the action tendency moves people to expand and thrust forward in order to set boundaries. However, anger itself is not a singular thing, but varies widely: it may only last a few minutes, or it can smoulder for days (even years); it can be hot and explosive, or cold and rejecting. The same goes for all emotions. Each is a theme with many variations, and these variations are important. A simple one-word emotion label is never enough to help us to fully appreciate what the emotion is trying to tell us about our situation or what is most useful to do about it.

Primary adaptive emotion responses. The most important distinction, however, is between the different functions of each type of emotion response. For example, anger may be an empowering adaptive response to being violated or a reactive blaming response to feeling hurt. The first kind of emotion response is a gut reaction that we call *primary adaptive*. Here, *primary* means 'first', not necessarily most important. Also, *adaptive* means 'useful'. A primary adaptive emotion response is our first, natural reaction to a current situation and helps us take appropriate action. We described a broad range of these in the previous section. They help cope with current situations and when the situation that produced them is dealt with or disappears, they fade. They are quick to arrive and fast to leave. All initial emotional reactions are primary emotions; however, not all primary emotions are adaptive, as we will shortly see.

Secondary reactive emotion responses. As we said, another kind of anger may be a blaming overreaction to a current situation, driven by an underlying feeling of shame. Although anger may be our immediate reaction, it often comes as a secondary response to an underlying, prior, and often implicit feeling. We have seen in our practice that in many cultures, men stereotypically express secondary reactive anger. They might actually be experiencing shame or fear, but because they believe that it is not manly to be afraid, they may instead respond by becoming angry. When emotions cover up other emotions in this way, we call them *secondary reactive emotion responses* (secondary emotions for short). Secondary emotions are reactions to primary emotions, or are feelings about primary emotions, that is, feelings about feelings. So, we might be angry as a response to feeling hurt, or feel guilty because we're angry at someone. Our secondary emotions serve a function, protecting us from feeling a distressing primary emotion. If something makes us feel sad and we get angry, we might push others away and thus avoid being asked about the sadness. However, our need for comfort is still there. Therefore, a crucial point about secondary emotions is that while being protective, they keep us from getting what we need. If we're feeling sad, but showing anger instead, we won't get comfort and support. If we're feeling angry, but showing sadness, people might still violate our boundaries.

Instrumental emotion responses. We may also express emotions intentionally or even unintentionally to get a desired result, such as crying to get sympathy. These are feelings expressed with the intent to influence others, independently of whether we actually feel them, often to get others to pay attention to us or to approve of us. Common examples include 'crocodile tears' (instrumental sadness), 'crying wolf' (instrumental fear), intimidation displays (instrumental anger), and faking unconditional positive regard when we don't feel it (instrumental compassion). These are learned expressive behaviours or experiences that we sometimes use to influence or manipulate others. The intention may be conscious or nonconscious. So David might cry intentionally to avoid his partner's anger, or Leo may grow automatically grouchy to scare away Penny, who is trying to get close to him, without being aware that he is doing this. This may come from a learned pattern in his childhood… or not.

Primary maladaptive emotion responses. These include habitual fear of insecurity or of danger, shame about inadequacy or the sadness of lonely abandonment, and are also a person's first, automatic reaction to a situation. These reactions in the present are overlearned responses from the past, based on previous traumatic experiences, failures by caregivers to help us regulate our emotional pain or experiences of abandonment, neglect or humiliation. These emotional responses may have been adaptive in the original situation but they are no longer helpful in the present. For example, clients may feel fear when their loving partners come close because of past hurt from parents' rejection or abuse. So these emotional responses are more a reflection of past unresolved issues than reactions to the present situation and they do not prepare the individual for adaptive action in the present. These feelings are still our most fundamental, 'true' feelings, but they are no longer 'healthy' feelings; instead, they are core emotional wounds. Debilitating fear, basic insecurity, the sadness of lonely abandonment, pervasive shame and humiliation, destructive rage, and unresolved grief are some of the most common examples of this category of emotions.

Maladaptive emotions are those old familiar feelings that we know well. They are like good old friends who are bad for us. We suffer a lot of pain and turmoil from them. We feel stuck in these emotions. Every time we sink into them, they make us feel just as bad as the last time. They can last long after the situation that caused them, staying with us for years as unhealed wounds. When these wounded states emerge, they seem to have a mind of their own. When they are evoked, we sink into them in inexplicable and helpless ways. These might be old, familiar feelings of longing and deprivation, anxious isolation, feeling worthless, being not good enough, or feeling inexplicably angry and blaming. These are the bad feelings that hold us prisoner and from which we so desperately want to escape. Such emotions are generally disorganizing. They do not suggest a clear sense of direction. Typically, they reveal more about us than about the situation.

An example of this type of emotion is exemplified by Jonah, who in session 3, when talking about his difficulties with his boss, says 'as soon as I walk into my boss's office I get this sinking feeling in my stomach'. His memory-based emotion schemes of his fear of his mother's criticisms combined with his past experience of his boss's dis approval guide his appraisals, bias his decisions, and generate his physical arousal and action tendency to want to escape. These emotion schemes, while having been adaptive as a child, are maladaptive for him now. When emotion schemes become problematic, like the fear-based schemes generating the sinking feeling in Jonah's stomach, they become important targets for therapeutic work (Greenberg & Paivio, 1997).

Maladaptive emotions can be basic ones, such as fear and shame, or more complex ones, such as Jonah's not yet articulated sinking feeling, or of other feelings he might have, such as feelings of empty isolation or lonely alienation. The most common and important maladaptive basic emotions that we have found in general counselling populations are fear/anxiety, sadness, and shame. It is helpful to note here two different types of maladaptive fear/anxiety: traumatic fear which comes from the fear of danger and leads us to run away from the danger; and fear of abandonment (attachment anxiety), which leads us to run towards the source of the fear. Each can be a core wound. Certain emotions tend to become maladaptive through *traumatic learning*, in which an originally adaptive emotion, such as appropriate fear of gunshots in battle, can become so deeply etched into our psyche that it becomes generalized to situations that are no longer dangerous, setting off alarms of danger when no danger is present. For example, we might duck for cover and relive horrifying scenes of war every time a car backfires. In such a case, emotions from the past are clearly intruding into the present. Often they are more subtle and lead to a feeling of lack of trust or a sense of inadequacy. Whatever they are, they disrupt close relationships and destroy our feelings of self-worth.

Thus, counsellors need to learn how to work with clients to help them identify what kinds of emotion response are operating, both in specific situations and more generally. This kind of shared emotion assessment then becomes the basis for a collaborative case formulation in EFC, which in turn guides what client and counsellor need to work on, as we discuss in the next chapter.

Further Exploration

Reading

Elliott, R., Watson, J. C., Goldman, R. N., & Greenberg, L. S. (2004). *Learning emotion-focused therapy: The process-experiential approach to change.* Washington, DC: American Psychological Association. [See Chapter 2]

Greenberg, L. S. (2019). Theory of functioning in emotion-focused therapy. In L. S. Greenberg & R. N. Goldman (Eds.), *Clinical handbook of emotion-focused therapy* (pp. 37–59). Washington, DC: American Psychological Association.

Greenberg, L. S., Rice, L. N., & Elliott, R. (1993). *Facilitating emotional change: The moment-by-moment process.* New York: Guilford Press.

Watching

Elliott, R. (2016). *Emotional Deepening Process.* The Counselling Channel. Online video available at: www.youtube.com/watch?v=kNRg2DFtgOw

Greenberg, L. S. (2016). *Leslie Greenberg on Emotion-Focused Therapy: From Certainty through Chaos to Complexity.* Psychotherapy Expert Talks. Online video available at: www.youtube.com/watch?v=rYvcLJcpghY&list=PLvSprSnWnWIf2di3o7DMZaNwTdhXprEqk&index=2&t=91s

Norwegian Institute of Emotion Focused Therapy (2015). *Alfred and Shadow: A Short Story about Emotions.* Animated video available at: www.youtube.com/watch?v=SJOjpprbfeE&feature=youtu.be

Reflecting

1. Can you think of a time when you got stuck in an emotion, a time when you couldn't get out of the emotion and you just kept going around in circles with it? What was it?
2. Now, can you think of a time when an emotion helped you move forward in your life (in other words, when it helped you get unstuck)? What was that?
3. Think of a time recently when you experienced a strong or striking emotional reaction. Now, see if you can use the emotion scheme model to elaborate the five components of this experience. (See pp. 24–27 and Figure 2.1 if you need help.)
4. See if you can identify examples from your own experience of each of the four main emotion response types. Write brief descriptions of each. (See pp. 35–37.)

3

Deepening and Transforming Emotion

Chapter Outline

Emotion Transformation and the Emotional Deepening Model

Entry Points into the Change Process

The Emotional Deepening Model in EFC

Conclusion

Further Exploration

Emotion Transformation and the Emotional Deepening Model

So how do EFC counsellors begin using the emotion theory that we presented in the previous chapter to help clients transform their problematic emotions into useful ones? The aim of EFC is to help clients to gently activate feelings related to problematic issues, in order to help them make sense of their emotions and transform them. This transformation process can be thought of in various ways:

- Changing emotion with emotion (for example, compassion transforms sadness; anger transforms fear; Greenberg, 2015);
- Working with the interplay (we call it a *dialectic*) between aspects of the person, including thought and feeling, to spark new emotional experience (Elliott & Greenberg, 1997; Greenberg et al., 1993); and
- Emotional deepening via a series of steps from more superficial, unproductive emotions to deeper, more productive emotions (see below).

Regardless of how we understand emotion transformation (see Greenberg, 2015, in press), we always have to start somewhere; we need entry points.

Entry Points into the Change Process

A good place to start is the crucial difference between talking about our emotions and directly experiencing them. The seventeenth-century French philosopher René Descartes said, 'I think, therefore I am'; in EFC we say, 'I feel, therefore I am'. In any significant personal experience, our feelings come first; our thoughts come later, sometimes much later. This means that in EFC we see people as wiser than their intellects alone, with emotion providing important, useful information about their situation and how to respond to it.

The main entry points in EFC are (a) therapist empathic attunement with client emotions, (b) focusing client attention on bodily feelings, and (c) experiments in directed awareness and emotion stimulation using imagery and psychodramatic enactments. All of these are used to focus on feeling. So EFC counsellors learn specific methods to help clients concentrate their attention on their as yet unsymbolized emotional experiences. This enables them to help their clients put their feelings into words, and to intensify the vividness of their experience so that they, the clients, can get what their emotions are trying to tell them. Once clients have arrived at their emotions, they either utilize them as guides or, if the emotions are painful, stuck ones that are no longer good guides, they can transform them with new emotional experiences.

These specific ways of focusing on emotion involve different ways of relating to clients rather than engaging in interventions to fix or modify clients. Methods of deepening experience are ways of relating facilitatively to help clients access their emotions and the organismic wisdom embedded in these emotions, and to transform them when they are no longer good guides. Clients are seen as experts on their experience. We help clients to access their own emotions. We agree with Rogers: 'It is the client who knows what hurts' (1961: 11); they know what is painful and has been disallowed. At the same time, we have found that clients can often benefit from help in accessing and accepting their emotions, and that this will help them identify what they need and what directions they need to take to heal. People are viewed as experts on their experience and as wiser than their intellects alone. Counsellors, on the other hand, are seen as experts on process facilitation, who help clients access and process their own emotions.

Furthermore, in EFC this holds true even for difficult, painful or stuck emotions that don't feel like they are helping. EFC works not only on accepting feelings but also on the principle that we cannot leave a place (or emotion) until we have arrived at it; for this reason, we encourage our clients to accept their emotions and to listen to the information these provide. However, once emotions have been arrived at, those that are painful and no longer useful, like certain forms of stuck fear, sadness and shame, also need to be transformed by accessing new emotions.

Where reason cannot penetrate, cognitive and psycho–educative methods that appeal to reason and deliberate processing will not work, and emotional change processes are needed. Change in the domain of amygdala-based emotions like fear requires both awareness of these old stuck emotions and their transformation. Awareness is facilitated by approaching and attending to the emotion, heightening and tolerating it, symbolizing it, most often in words, and becoming aware of the things that trigger it. Transformation occurs by activating problematic maladaptive emotions and both experiencing new emotions and working with opposing action tendencies through an emotional deepening process; this then enables clients to construct new narrative meanings to consolidate change into a new personal narrative.

The Emotional Deepening Model in EFC

The past 20 years has seen the emergence of a general model of the emotion deepening and transformation process in EFC (e.g., Greenberg, 2015; Pascual-Leone & Greenberg, 2007; Timulak, 2015). This model pulls together much of what we have been saying in this and the previous chapter and is summarized in Table 3.1.

TABLE 3.1 *Emotion transformation: The emotional deepening model in EFC*

Emotion Process/Stage	What the Counsellor Generally Does
A. Pre-Deepening Work	(Address these before moving into Main Deepening Sequence)
A-1. Instrumental ('fake' emotions)	If these cause problems for the counselling work, explore them with the client in order to understand the interpersonal intention behind them.
A-2. Overwhelmed-dysregulated	Help client to moderate: offer empathic understanding, empathic affirmation; use various brief or longer forms of emotion moderation work.
B. Main Deepening Sequence	(Most of counselling involves this)
B-1. Interrupted-shut-down-restricted	Help client to explore and resolve self-interruption processes and other ways of restricting their emotions (externalizing, dwelling on body symptoms, going into their heads, and impulsive leaping into action).
B-2. Undifferentiated/unclear emotion ['bad']	Accept, explore, and help client to differentiate.
B-3. Presenting emotion symptoms: Secondary Reactive	Offer empathy and help client to explore in order to find the implicit primary emotions that come before/ underneath.

(Continued)

TABLE 3.1 *(Continued)*

Emotion Process/Stage	What the Counsellor Generally Does
B-4. Old stuck bad feelings: Primary Maladaptive 1	Offer empathy and help client to explore and deepen to identify the core pain ('what hurts the most').
B-5. Core pain: Primary Maladaptive 2 → unmet need	Validate and provide empathic affirmation of core pain and what it needs.
B-6. Primary Adaptive: connecting sadness, assertive anger, self-compassion	Help client to stay with, receive and appreciate the emerging useful feelings and the useful information they contain.
C. Post-Deepening Work	(Happens primarily at the end of tasks or sessions)
Creating a Meaning Perspective	Help client to step back and reflect on the emotion work that has been done; create new narrative meaning; 'connect the head and the heart'.

The latest version of this model, presented here, has three phases: pre-deepening work, the main deepening sequence, and post-deepening work.

A. Pre-deepening work. Emotional deepening requires safety, both in the counselling relationship and within the client. It's useful to distinguish two kinds of pre-deepening work, addressing instrumental emotion responses and dealing with overwhelmed dys-regulation.

A-1. Instrumental. In the first place, it is difficult for our clients to access their emotions if they are too worried about what the counsellor thinks of them, or if they feel like they have to perform for us to get their needs met. In this situation, our clients will be focused on using emotions instrumentally, for example, to impress us with their need for counselling, or to get us to feel sorry for them or to see them as good people; sometimes, they may even be trying to intimidate us or make us feel guilty. When these processes interfere significantly with counselling or when they annoy or frustrate us as counsellors, it becomes necessary for us to attend to this first before doing anything else. Usually, this can be done by having a conversation with the client about how the counselling is going for them, especially what they are hoping for from us, and what we might be doing that could be getting in their way. (In EFC, this is a task that we call *relational dialogue*; see Chapter 5, Table 5.1.)

A-2. Overwhelmed-dysregulated. The other time when we need to do pre-deepening work with clients is when they are emotionally dysregulated in the sense of feeling overwhelmed, as we discussed in Chapter 2. In EFC, emotion regulation is a *meta-task*, a kind of overarching task that runs across various kinds of therapeutic in-session work. Table 3.2 gives examples of a range of different kinds of emotion moderation work in EFC, listed in order of increasing process guiding. In working with a panicky or severely overwhelmed client, the counsellor may offer a blend of several different emotion moderation strategies.

TABLE 3.2 *Examples of emotion moderation work in EFC*

Support and empathy:

- Counsellor offers genuine empathic understanding and unconditional positive regard
- Empathic affirmation/prizing voice (Gently: 'I can see how difficult this has been for you.')

Symbolizing painful emotion:

- Represent client painful experience in words or images (e.g., 'It's like there's this a crack down the middle of you, and there's no bottom to it.')

Containing language/imagery:

- Use summing up/formulating responses ('So those are some of the main issues here.')
- Reflect using 'it' or 'something' ('Something in you hurts.')

Small pieces of emotion moderation work:

- Help client to attain a useful working distance ('Can you imagine taking that pain about your son and pushing away from you for now?')
- Help client to imagine a safe space ('Can you imagine a place where you feel safe? Maybe a favourite place? Now, can you imagine going into your safe space and let yourself feel that?')
- Grounding/mindfulness work ('Maybe say hello to something in you that's scared?')

Emotion-moderating therapeutic tasks (see Chapter 5, Table 5.1):

- Clearing a Space (a kind of Focusing)
- Empathic Affirmation for Vulnerability
- Meaning Creation for Meaning Protest
- Compassionate Self-soothing for Anguish
- Psychological Contact Work for dissociation, panic or psychotic states

B. Main Deepening Sequence. Just as most stars (including our sun) follow a common path of stellar evolution, most of EFC involves helping clients to move themselves from more surface-level, less productive emotions to deeper, more useful emotions. In the middle section of Table 3.1 we describe a series of six steps, from restricted to primary adaptive.

B-1. Interrupted-shut-down-restricted. Often clients enter counselling with their emotions quite blocked or restricted. Clients in depressed states typically feel blocked or stuck; clients who have been traumatized frequently feel numb or cut off not only from trauma-related emotions like fear, but from all emotions. As we noted in Chapter 2, such clients are suffering from an emotion regulation difficulty: they are *over-regulated*. This over-regulation may take the form of a general pattern of emotional restriction in which the person habitually attends *away* from their emotions, to external events, to bodily complaints, to intellectualizing, or into action. Or it may appear in the session in the form of *self-interruption*, a kind of internal conflict in which the person starts to feel something, then stops themselves (for more on kinds of internal conflicts and working with self-interruption, see Chapter 6). Obviously, when the client is self-interrupting or restricting their emotions, it is going to be difficult to proceed, so the counsellor will need to attend to this process first before going further. (See Greenberg & Woldarsky Meneses, 2019; and Paivio & Pascual-Leone, 2010, for useful and detailed accounts of working self-interruption in work with clients with complex trauma and emotional injuries.)

B-2. Undifferentiated/unclear emotions. Even if the client doesn't start counselling in a state of emotional restriction or self-interruption, they often begin with undifferentiated or non-specific emotions. You ask them what they are feeling, and they say, 'bad', 'stressed' or 'frustrated'. When this happens, we accept the undifferentiated experience and help the client explore and describe the feeling: 'Bad... You just feel bad inside... Can you say more? ... What kind of 'bad' is it?' Or maybe, 'What do you feel bad about?' This also applies when the client offers a simple one-word emotion label, like 'sad' or 'angry'. The counsellor asks the client to try to specify what kind of sad or angry they are feeling. In EFC, a single-word emotion label is never enough to properly describe and understand what we are feeling.

B-3. Presenting emotion symptoms: Secondary Reactive. Once they have been differentiated, the client's more specific initial presenting emotion symptoms (such as depression, worry, social anxiety, angry outbursts) emerge, and it often turns out that these are secondary reactive emotion responses, as we described in the previous chapter. In other words, they are a reaction such as hopelessness to another more primary emotion, such as fear (anger and shame are also common). Even though it is secondary, it is still what the client is feeling at the moment, so it's important to offer empathy to these secondary feelings. As we say in EFC: 'You have to arrive at an emotion before you can leave it.' As we help the client to explore it, we begin to hear, first, the mismatch between the situation and the emotion, and, second, a hint of another emotion underneath or before the presenting emotion symptom. This could be yet another secondary emotion, part of a longer chain of secondary reactive emotions. Most often, however, the underlying prior emotion is primary: the person's first, direct response to the situation.

B-4. Old stuck bad feelings: Primary Maladaptive 1. Sometimes our clients' presenting difficulties are primary maladaptive emotion responses, such as chronic anger based on repeated experiences of abuse, or familiar depression stemming from a history of neglect or abandonment. However, much of the time with our clients, we only get to the old, familiar stuck feelings after first exploring their presenting secondary emotion symptoms. Examples include:

- Unresolved resentment at a parent that is behind the depression.
- Underlying shame about being defective that makes us afraid of other people (= social anxiety). As we will see, this arises for both of our running case examples: in Jonah's case from the maltreatment by his mother, and in Bethany's case from being treated as a harmful person by both of her parents.
- Guilty over-responsibility that leads us to worry all the time in order to prevent disaster, which is common in clients with generalized anxiety, which is often based in childhood insecurity (see Timulak & McElvaney, 2017; Watson & Greenberg, 2017).

Helping a client get to the primary maladaptive emotion is important progress for clients, but it typically doesn't leave them feeling better; in fact, they may feel worse, because now they feel the pain from which they had been protecting themselves; now they know how and why they feel so stuck. It's important to offer empathy and help clients explore these old bad stuck emotions; however, this is not going to be enough to help them get unstuck and move forward. Instead, what is needed is to realize that there are multiple layers of primary maladaptive emotions. There is another layer and a further step of deepening that is essential for helping clients to transform their primary maladaptive emotions. In order to help the client move forward and get unstuck, the therapist helps the client use the *emotion compass* (e.g., in empty chair work, see Chapter 7) by asking the client, 'What hurts the most in all of this?', or 'When you think about your dad, what do you most miss?' (or resent, feel guilty about, etc.). This helps the client both to differentiate and to heighten the painful emotion, as it takes the client to the core wound.

B-5. Core pain: Primary Maladaptive 2. Helping our clients fully arrive at their core pain is an important turning point in EFC, and occurs across a wide range of therapeutic tasks, as we shall see in Chapters 5–8. When this happens, it is vital for us to let ourselves empathically resonate with the deep vulnerability associated with our clients' core pain. This enables us to feel genuine compassion for the client. Instrumental compassion will not do; most clients will be able to tell that we are faking it. We have to really let our client's pain touch us, feel the compassion, and speak from it, providing empathic affirmation and validating the client at this deepest level. By asking about core pain, we help the client to go past the stuckness of the primary maladaptive emotion response to universal, existential human truths: our vulnerability, fragility, loneliness, fear of abandonment, uncertainty about our value to ourselves, and others. We ask them what is truly most important in their life. Then, once we are sure that the client really has hit bottom, and once we have let them know honestly and directly that we are there with them, then we can ask them about the need associated with the core pain: 'This feeling that hurts the most, … what does it need?'

B-6. Primary Adaptive. The answer to the question of what the core pain needs is a universal human need; it is something that we all need: empathy, acknowledgement, validation, connection, protection, compassion. Not only do we need it, we also deserve it, even (or especially!) when it's missing. It is part of our human and evolutionary birthright. Experiencing the counsellor's compassion and validation helps the client to experience their core pain's need as real and valid, and this other- and self-validation transforms primary maladaptive core pain into an adaptive emotion, most commonly: connecting sadness, assertive anger, or self-compassion. When this happens, the counsellor helps the client to stay with and appreciate the emerging primary adaptive emotion and the useful information that it contains. This new emotion changes the old emotion as when assertive anger transforms shame and the client ends up feeling a sense of pride or worthiness.

C. Post-deepening work: Creating a Meaning Perspective. As we have been saying, emotion work is not complete until the client is able to step back out of the intensity of their emotions and reflect on them, while still staying grounded in them. This is the point in the work where client and counsellor collaborate to help the client create a meaning perspective, to formulate a new narrative or story about how the client's process works and where that leaves them. As we will illustrate in later chapters, this formulation will also point the way forward to the next steps in counselling or beyond it.

Conclusion

The EFC deepening and transforming process is complex and we have presented here a model of phases to help explain how it works. Of course, people and their processes are complex and multifaceted and so this is a simplification of human complexity. It is, however, a guide to provide a picture of the steps or phases of the change process. Hopefully as you read the following chapters it will flesh this out and help you get a feel for how it all works. The main take-home points are presented in Table 3.3, along with some of our favourite EFC sayings, all written in easy-to-understand client language. You can even print these take-home points out and give them to your clients to take home with them!

TABLE 3.3 *Information for clients about emotion-focused counselling*

Why Emotions are Important and How We Get Stuck in Them

- **Three reasons why emotions are important:**

  1. *They tell us what is <u>important</u> to us.*
  2. *They tell us what we need or want, and that helps us figure out what to <u>do</u>.*
  3. *They give us a sense of consistency and <u>wholeness</u>.*

- **Four main ways to get stuck in emotions:**

  1. *Let our emotions get out of balance*: Sometimes the level of emotion is *too much* or *too little*.
  2. *Use other emotions to cover up the most useful emotions*: The most important or helpful emotion is sometimes *underneath* the most obvious emotion.
  3. *Ignore important aspects of our emotions*: Sometimes we get stuck in an emotion because we're *missing* an important *piece* of it.
  4. *Get stuck in emotions left over from previous bad experiences*: Sometimes our response to a present situation might be more about things that happened in the past.

- **Some EFC sayings:**

  ○ You have to arrive at an emotion before you can leave it.
  ○ The thing that hurts the most points to what is most important.
  ○ The head and the heart need each other.
  ○ Emotion is what connects us to each other.
  ○ Every feeling has a need, and every need has a direction for action.

Further Exploration

Reading

Goldman, R., & Greenberg, L. S. (2014). *Case formulation in emotion-focused therapy*. Washington, DC: American Psychological Association.

Greenberg, L. S. (2016). *Emotion focused therapy: Theory and practice* (2nd ed.). Washington, DC: American Psychological Association.

Greenberg, L. S., & Goldman R. (2019). Theory of practice. In L. S. Greenberg & R. N. Goldman (Eds.), *Clinical handbook of emotion-focused therapy* (pp. 61–90). Washington, DC: American Psychological Association.

Timulak, L. (2015). *Transforming emotional pain in psychotherapy: An emotion-focused approach.* Hove, East Sussex: Routledge.

Watching

Elliott, R. (2016). *Understanding Emotion-Focused Therapy with Robert Elliott.* Counselling Channel Videos, Glastonbury, UK. Online video available at: https://vimeo.com/ondemand/understandingeft/167235549

Greenberg, L. S. (2020). *Six Principles for Working with Emotions.* Counselling Channel, Glastonbury, UK. Online video available at: www.youtube.com/watch?v=VfsVqk-ke_s

Timulak, L. (2020). *Transforming Emotional Pain: An Illustration of Emotion-Focused Therapy.* Counselling Channel, Glastonbury, UK. Online video available at: www.youtube.com/watch?v=d63-dJcilrE&t=53s

Reflecting

1. Think of a time when you have had an emotion and then it changed. What happened?
2. For discussion: If we have a model of how clients can deepen and transform their maladaptive emotions, what are the implications for counsellors? How much do you think counsellors should push their clients to deepen their emotions?
3. See if you can focus on a painful memory from your past:

   • As you remember it, focus on what happens in your body. Take your time. When the feeling comes, see if you can name it.
   • Ask yourself what in the feeling hurt the most. See what comes.
   • After this, ask the part of the feeling that hurt the most what it (and you) needed in the situation.
   • See what you feel now in the light of this need. Is it a new healthier feeling that helps you transform what you feel?

4

Beginning Emotion-Focused Counselling: Fostering the Relationship and Beginning the Work

Chapter Outline

The Opening Phase of Emotion-Focused Counselling

Empathic Attunement to Emotion and Types of Empathic Response in EFC

Establishing Therapeutic Presence

Actively Collaborating with the Client and Beginning to Develop a Shared Case Formulation

Initial Narrative Work: Helping the Client to Tell Their Story

Jonah Begins Counselling

Further Exploration

The Opening Phase of Emotion-Focused Counselling

In this chapter we describe the opening phase of EFC, during which client and counsellor get to know each other and begin their therapeutic journey. As we've seen in Chapter 3, the most important feature of this journey is helping the client begin to pay attention to their emotions and put them into words so that they can deepen them. In order for the client to transform old stuck emotions into productive, useful emotions they must experience the things in their life that hurt the most (*core pain*). Clearly, this process depends on the counsellor deeply understanding the client, and on the client trusting the counsellor to a high degree. How does the counsellor help the client begin this difficult work, letting themselves experience the very feelings that they most want to turn away from? The answer to this dilemma can be found in the three key relationship principles we described in Chapter 1: the counsellor's deep empathic attunement, their strong therapeutic presence, and their active collaboration with the client. In the early sessions of EFC, the main work for client and counsellor is building a safe, productive therapeutic relationship strong enough to sustain the difficult work ahead. In other words, the relationship is the first task of counselling: *alliance formation*. Table 4.1 presents the stages of this alliance formation task, including common difficulties at each point.

TABLE 4.1   *Stages of the alliance formation task in EFC*

Alliance Formation Process	Common Difficulties
(1. *Marker*: Client begins therapy)	(Client drops out before first session)
2. *Initiating*: Empathic attunement; initiating a safe working environment; establishing therapeutic presence (emotional connection of acceptance and openness)	Client feels misunderstood, judged, or unsafe; regards therapist as insincere or untrustworthy; perceives empathic attunement as a dangerous intrusion
3. *Locating therapeutic focus*: Developing a sense of what is significant or central for the client (therapist's inner sense, knowledge of functioning; client's sense of what is important; explicit client questions; foci of attention; task markers)	Absence of therapeutic focus; client has difficulty finding and maintaining a focus, is scattered or generally defers to therapist
4. *Partial resolution: Goal agreement*: Establishing agreement on therapeutic foci or goals	Client ambivalent about change, not firmly committed to working towards goals related to main therapeutic focus; sees the causes of their problems differently from therapist
5. *Task agreement*: Establishing agreement on how to work toward therapeutic goals (beginning to engage in empathic exploration, addressing emergent client concerns about task)	Client has difficulty turning attention inward; questions the purpose and value of engaging in therapy to deal with problems; has expectations about tasks and process that diverge from those of therapist
6. *Full resolution: Productive working environment*: Client trusts therapist, engages actively in productive therapeutic work	

And, yes, along the way, client and counsellor are also going to begin the process of digging around the client's presenting difficulties (*empathic exploration*), and of course the client is going to want to unfold the story of how they got to this point (*narrative retelling*). Table 4.2 summarizes the main tasks within the opening phase of EFC.

TABLE 4.2 *Main tasks of the opening phase of emotion-focused counselling*

Task Marker	Therapeutic Work	Key Change Point
Beginning of counselling: Client walks in the door	*Alliance Formation*: Engaging the client in the work of therapy	*Achieving a productive working environment*: Client trusts counsellor and actively engages in productive therapeutic work
Problem-relevant Experience: Client expresses personal interest in an experience that is powerful, troubling, incomplete, too general, abstract, or expressed only in external terms	*Empathic Exploration*: Helping client to turn attention to internal experience and re-experience past events; help them to search the edges, specify, and elaborate those experiences	*Clarification*: Client experiences some clarification of the experience; clear marker for a more specific task may emerge (e.g., conflict split)
Narrative Pressure: Client displays internal pressure to tell story of difficult event (e.g., trauma, presenting difficulty)	*Narrative Retelling*: Help client to tell story of difficult event, including re-experiencing of specific details of external events, inner experiences and meanings	*Critical point*: Client spells out and re-experiences the most difficult moment(s) in their story

Empathic Attunement to Emotion and Types of Empathic Response in EFC

Why empathy is so important in EFC. Many people think that EFC is all about the furniture: two chair work for negative treatment of self ('conflict splits') and empty chair work for unresolved relationship issues ('unfinished business'). In fact, we will devote most of Chapters 6 and 7 to these tasks. However, there is a secret ingredient in EFC, something that makes it all work, especially the chair work: deep *empathic attunement with client emotion*. If you treat EFC as a bag of tricks, as all about the active tasks, you will fail. You will go into your head, lose empathy, and your use of EFC tasks will be awkward, out of tune with your client, and won't go anywhere. If you are lucky, your client will not really engage in the therapeutic work and you will feel ineffective; if you (and your client) are unlucky, they will quit therapy, leaving with a kind of interpersonal allergy to working with painful emotions and talking to furniture. You will have failed your client, yourself, and even their next counsellor, who will be stuck dealing with the allergy.

For this reason, empathic attunement is a big deal in EFC, important enough that we prefer to use a slightly different term for it: instead of empathy, plain and simple, we are going to talk about *empathic attunement*, and are going to emphasize emotion in discussing it here in its richness and complexity. Empathic attunement is the first and most important of the six principles of EFC practice that we described in Chapter 1.

In our experience, learning EFC puts great demands on your empathy skills; you are more likely to struggle with blocks to your empathy than with the technical skills of facilitating chair work. We have often found this to be the case with counsellors from other forms of counselling, even person-centred counsellors. EFC asks you not just to communicate that you understand your client's main message or point (their meaning), but to tune into your client's emotional experience with high precision, getting it as accurately as possible and tracking it as it changes from moment to moment in the session. EFC also asks you to communicate your empathic attunement in a vivid, evocative manner, to use your body (not your head) to guess what is hovering at the edge of the client's experience, especially their emotions, and to do so with a kind of firm tentativeness marked with humility and genuine curiosity. Most critically, when your client accesses vulnerability or emotional pain, EFC asks you to let your client's pain resonate with your pain and asks you to lean into that mutual pain, to stay with it, and to express it to your client with compassion and courage.

A bit more brain theory. Modern social neuroscience (Decety & Ickes, 2009) has shown that empathy has three key components, which are also linked to specific parts of the human brain. First, there is an automatic, intuitive *emotional resonance* process that mirrors the emotional elements of the other person's bodily experience. This process is experienced primarily in your throat/chest/stomach area and is based mostly in an older part of the human brain called the limbic system (Decety & Lamm, 2009). We can tell what is going on in our limbic system because it talks to the trunk of our bodies, which we can call 'heart' for short. Most of us are born with this ability, although in growing up we were probably taught to ignore it. In EFC, we just have to let ourselves access this innate capacity instead of ignoring it, although in some cases, we may have to re-learn it.

Second, there is a more deliberate *perspective-taking* process, particularly located in newer parts of our brains (prefrontal and temporal cortex; Shamay-Tsoory, 2009). This aspect of empathy involves actively imagining being the client, and it can be hard work, but the upside is that we get to use our heads as well as our hearts to do this.

Third, there is an *emotion-regulation* process that we use to soothe our distress when we let ourselves feel the other person's pain. This process allows us to step back a bit and calm our emotional pain at our client's emotional pain; this helps us stay with it so that we can find our compassion and use it to offer help to our clients (this is probably based in other newer parts of our brain, specifically the orbitofrontal, prefrontal and parietal cortex; Decety & Lamm, 2009).

Practising body metaphors for empathy. The point of all this brain theory is not to reduce empathy to brain processes but to point out that as human beings we are evolved with the capacity for empathy, which EFC builds on and tries to deepen. In general, deepening our empathic attunement to client emotion requires personal development work, building the courage we discussed in Chapter 1 and working on anything that blocks our ability to tune into our own and others' emotions. Brain theory is fine and sounds very scientific, but we think that a better place to begin accessing and developing your empathy can be found in the formula in Table 4.3. When you have a chance and are on your own, take a few minutes to practise the empathic movements and accompanying symbolic bodily gestures, which are physical metaphors for what empathy feels like in EFC.

TABLE 4.3   *To be fully empathic, I need to...*

Empathic Movement	Symbolic Bodily Gesture
1. *Let go* of my personal issues, worries, distractions, and preconceptions about the client.	Make a fist; turn your hand palm up; open your hands and arms while imagining letting go of your pre-occupations and waiting for what the other has to offer. (This can be helped by taking a few minutes for yourself before your client arrives, in order to identify any lingering issues and to imagine setting them to one side.)
2. *Enter* my client's experience, like coming in their front door.	Raise both of your hands so that they are level in front of you, with palms facing down; move them forward, lowering them about six inches as you do so; maybe duck your head also while imagining ducking under the doorway of a small house.
3. *Resonate* with my client's experience, like being a human tuning fork, finding what in my experience responds to their experience.	Raise both of your hands in front of you so that your fingers are pointing up and roughly parallel to each other; imagine them vibrating in tune with a sound, perhaps pulsing gently.
4. *Search* for what feels most poignant, central, important in the client's immediate experience.	Imagine that you are standing in front of a table with a jumble of bits and pieces spread out on it, as if you had dumped out the contents of your purse, sewing kit or change jar on the table; now move your downward-facing, spread-out fingers around on the imaginary table as you search for just the right bit of something that you are looking for. (You will know it when you find it!)
5. *Grasp and express* this important experience by focusing in on it, finding words for it, and communicating it back to the client.	Close your hands on the imagined piece, grasping it in your fists; then turn your fists face up and move them forward, offering what you have grasped to the other, finally opening your fists and letting your offering go to the other.
Then return to Step 1: Let go again	Open your hands and arms to what comes next.

Empathic understanding responses in EFC. We're worried about starting our discussion of empathy in EFC by listing a bunch of different kinds of response, because we're afraid that you will end up trying to 'do empathy' as a technique, when it's really an attitude. If, however, you've got your head (and heart) around the attitude, we hope it will be safe for us to tell you about some of the many different ways you can be empathic in EFC. We'll do this in batches, starting with responses that are just about empathy and virtually nothing else, which we introduced in Chapter 1 as *empathic understanding* responses. EFC distinguishes between several different kinds of empathic understanding response. First, when you use *empathic reflections* you are listening for the main thing the client is trying to say, the key meaning or feeling. It could be about someone else (*third party reflection*), or about something they did or thought (*content reflection*), but ideally, it's about what they experienced or felt (*empathic reflection*) in a situation. For example, 15 minutes into Bethany's first session, the following exchange happened (empathic understanding responses in italics):

Segment 4-1 (15 min from start):

Bethany: Yeah, things will get to a point and then I'm so anxious about something, like, preoccupied by it, I can't really think of anything else.

Robert: *So it (your social anxiety) will just keep coming up and you'll be occupied by thinking of it.* And what kinds of things do you think about?

Bethany: Like of people coming over to the house, what are they going to think about the house and stuff. And it's like, what are people going to expect of me?, what am I supposed to do?

Robert: Uhuh, it's like you're kind of running a model in your head?

Bethany: Exactly.

Robert: *So wondering what exactly is going to happen, trying to imagine as vividly as possible.*

Bethany: Yeah, I try to imagine every single scenario. But you can't do that.

Here the therapist is mostly trying to track the main thing the client is saying, as accurately as possible, just as in traditional person-centred counselling.

The therapist also uses *empathic following* responses: brief acknowledgements or gentle word-for-word repetitions of what the client is saying. For example, in Segment 4-2, a bit later in the session, Bethany is talking about her relationship with her husband (empathic following responses in italics):

Segment 4-2 (about 35 min from start):

Bethany: Like I want to give him more, but I don't have any more to give.

Robert: I can't find it in me, *right* (done with a helpless, anxious voice and shoulder shrug).

Bethany: Yeah, because sometimes it upsets him as well, so then I feel bad about that.

Robert: *It upsets him*, he feels left out or outside (C: Yeah) or excluded.

Bethany: Yeah, exactly, he feels (pause) like I'm distant from him, I guess, [T: *yeah, cut off and distant*) and he doesn't want to, [T: *mhm*] so then that makes me feel bad.

In these brief responses the therapist is simply letting the client know that they are tracking what she is saying, as she gradually moves towards a more personal, painful topic.

As the client arrives at painful emotions, it's very important for the therapist to allow themselves to empathically resonate with the client's pain, and to express that, using *empathic affirmation* responses (italicized here):

Segment 4-2, continued:

Robert: Because you can see it hurts him, (C: mhm) and (gently:) it hurts you to see that, it causes some pain, or you might feel guilty about it (C: mhm), so then you want to be able to be more open. (C: Exactly) And

> I can imagine, of course, you can feel like you let him down, but (hesi-
> tantly:) also not good enough?
> *Bethany:* Yeah, often I feel that.

This passage shows how EFT therapists carefully, gently, but persistently help clients to move towards their emotions and especially their *core pain*, in this case the thing that hurts the most in interactions with other people. The key point here is that when the pain comes, it's essential for the therapist to lean into the pain, to face it with compassion, providing a kind of emotional holding of the client's raw, vulnerable feelings.

Empathic exploration responses in EFC. You have probably noticed that these two segments contain more than just empathic understanding responses. Other kinds of responses were happening also. For example, in Segment 4-1, the therapist asks an *exploratory question* in the second part of his first response: 'And what kinds of things do you think about?' These open questions are offered to help the client bring their experience to life by providing rich detail, as Bethany does in her next response. If you've had previous counselling training, it might surprise you to learn that these kinds of questions are perfectly OK in EFC; the important thing is to make sure that you reflect the client's answer to the question, as the therapist does by saying: 'It's like you're running a model in your head.' This is another kind of empathic exploration response, called an *empathic formulation*, in which the therapist is taking what the client has said and translating it into somewhat more technical language ('running a model in your head'), while making sure to accurately represent with the client has said.

Then, in the first response in Segment 4-2, the therapist does something interesting: they speak in the first person, as if they are the client ('I can't find it in me'). Such *evocative reflections* reflect the client's experience in a more vivid manner; often they are presented in a dramatic manner, such as the helpless voice and shoulder shrug that the therapist uses here. Evocative reflections often use vivid images or metaphors, such as when the therapist earlier in the session helped the client elaborate her metaphor of her social anxiety as a bomb:

Segment 4-3 (shortly before Segment 4-1):

> *Bethany:* So like, if my daughter and I are going to a playgroup or something like that, I'll always be apprehensive about that beforehand. But not like full-blown, anxious, (T: Uhuh) but apprehensive, it's like mild.
> *Robert:* Mild. That's like the fuse burning (C: Mhm) But then when it's full-blown, that's like the bomb going off? (C: yeah)

There are many different kinds of empathic exploration responses in EFC; however, two other important ones are exploratory reflections and empathic conjectures. *Exploratory reflections* are done in a tentative manner that encourages the client to explore further, while *empathic conjectures* are guesses about unexpressed feelings that the client might be having. Often, these go together, as in Segment 4-2 when the therapist says: 'And I can imagine, of course, you can feel like you let him down, but (hesitantly:) also not good enough?' Note how the therapist expresses tentativeness, using phrases like 'I can imagine', but also a hesitant, careful manner and a gentle, questioning tone. This helps the therapist go beyond the client's words to her possible unexpressed painful feelings. (Remember that we said this same response was also an empathic affirmation response.)

You might be wondering at this point, how you can learn to use all these different empathic understanding and empathic exploration responses in an effective manner. Here is a set of suggestions:

1. Start with an attitude of empathic attunement (see Table 4.3).
2. As you listen to your client, use your body to resonate with their feelings.
3. Do your best to put what resonates in your body into words that capture your client's feelings.
4. Record your sessions and listen back to them, paying particular attention to your client's immediate response to your empathic response.
5. Practise, practise, practise.

Establishing Therapeutic Presence

Empathy is also key to how EFC counsellors begin to build a strong, safe therapeutic alliance. In EFC, the client–counsellor relationship has two helpful functions (Rice, 1983). First, it helps create a sense of safety within the frame of the counselling, and this allows the client to open up and approach their emotional pain through the various kinds of emotion work offered in EFC. Second, a genuine, caring, empathic counselling relationship is healing in its own right, because it offers the client a corrective emotional experience.

The emotional labour of alliance formation. Empathic attunement is key, but the process of building a productive therapeutic relationship in EFC really begins with the therapist being very present with the client. This requires the counsellor to actively engage the client from the point of first contact (including on the telephone or in the email to make the initial appointment). This presence and engagement cannot be communicated by technique alone but must be firmly based on the counsellor's mindful, emotional stance with the client (Geller & Greenberg, 2012). In particular, the counsellor makes time to reach inside in order to access a mix of helpful emotions that motivate them to approach and engage with the client: in particular, curiosity, love (unconditional positive regard), and compassion. These emotions help the counsellor to be fully present with the client, even in composing emails.

First, however, we must address any internal interfering factors. We might be anxious about meeting a new person, or about our performance as a counsellor. We might be preoccupied with technique ('doing') rather than presence ('being'). We might have preconceptions about the client that are getting in our way, such as concerns based on what we have read in their intake file or differences in culture, age, sexual orientation and so on. Or there might be personal or work-related issues going on in our lives that are distracting us. The point is not to banish all these sorts of internal interferences. We are only human after all! Attacking these feelings, or ourselves for having them, will only distract us further. Instead, it's important to be aware of them and attempt to gently set them aside.

Sometimes all they need is a bit of understanding and a promise to come back to them in our next supervision session. (The Letting Go exercise from Table 4.3 can help also.)

Getting interfering factors out of the way, or at least putting them on hold for the time being, will make space for a range of helpful emotions that can support us in being present with our clients ('approach emotions'). Interest/curiosity helps us open up to the client and attend to them carefully, especially if it is not too clinical or distanced. A yearning for contact with others, perhaps driven partly by our own loneliness, can also be a resource, at least as long as it is well regulated and not too needy: here is another person to get to know, who brings with them a whole world of experience! A sense of ease stemming from inner freedom, or even joy in the work of counselling, can also be very helpful and can help us free up our playfulness and creativity. Finally, because we never know what is going to happen with each new person, courage to face the unknown is an important resource for EFC counsellors to cultivate.

Ways of being present with new clients. We have been saying that EFC involves both *being* and *doing*. It's not enough to focus on being emotionally present with clients; we also have to allow ourselves to show our being. In other words, we are involved in 'doing being' (Cowie, 2014). What does this look like? For the most part, presence is conveyed nonverbally, by our bodies and how we express ourselves in speaking:

- Appropriate eye contact: neither averting your gaze nor a fixed or piercing stare;
- Responsive facial expression that shows interest and at times matches the client's or the content of what they are talking about;
- Friendly manner, including allowing yourself to smile in response to jokes by the client, or in sympathy with what they are struggling to put across;
- Gentle, warm voice quality in response to client distress;
- Conveying by our manner that we are tolerant of our own and others' limitations;
- Allowing ourselves to reveal nonverbally when we feel touched or impacted by what the client is saying or feeling;
- And so on … (the list is open-ended)

Self-disclosure. Beginning counsellors often wonder if it is OK for them to disclose aspects of their experience to clients. The answer, as always, is 'it depends'. In EFC, counsellor self-disclosure is never an end in itself but is always done for a specific therapeutic reason. Most often, it is used to show empathy or caring, or to build or repair the therapeutic relationship. The example from the beginning of Chapter 1 is worth repeating here for emphasis. At the very beginning of her first session, in fact, while the therapist is setting up the camera, the client asks:

Bethany: Where are you from?

Robert: (realizing that she is trying to take the focus off herself, he smiles to himself:) So you want to know a bit about me. From my accent you'll be able to tell that I'm American, but I've been in Scotland for 10 years. (They sit down, he turns on the recorder.) I've been doing counselling for a while, but that doesn't stop me from being a bit nervous when I start with a new person. I wonder what you're experiencing, right now, as we start counselling?

This example illustrates several kinds of therapeutic presence. There is the slight smile that communicates that the therapist understands but isn't bothered that the client is deflecting attention from herself. Then they offer an informational *personal disclosure*, revealing a couple of general facts about self ('American', 'I've been doing counselling for a while'). This is followed by a deeper or more intimate *process disclosure* about feeling 'a bit nervous' at that moment in the session. In doing this, they model openness for the client, encouraging her to open up as well.

Actively Collaborating with the Client and Beginning to Develop a Shared Case Formulation

Locating the main therapeutic focus. In addition to strongly valuing counsellor empathic attunement and presence, EFC sees counselling as organized around therapeutic work on the client's difficult or painful experiences. Clients often present their problems in terms of symptoms, such as depression, anxiety or substance misuse. However, in EFC we are more interested in what hurts in the person's life. What important life project or goal is at risk, confronting them with the very real possibility that their life itself is going to be a failure? Is it having a satisfying, safe intimate relationship with a partner? Having kids and/or a career or meaningful work? Leaving the world a better place? What does the client feel is most significant or central for them to work on in counselling? Client presentations like depression, anxiety and so on are often the result of this hurt; but they may also be the cause of further injury, or at least make it worse. Working with the client to identify the main therapeutic focus is the first step in developing a *shared case formulation* (more on that shortly).

Note that the counsellor does not impose this *therapeutic focus* on the client. It is the *client's* sense of what hurts the most that matters, although the client may have trouble at first putting this into words, and the counsellor may have some sense of where the pain comes from, which they can offer tentatively to the client. The question is, how does the counsellor help the client locate their main therapeutic focus?

The simple answer is: *provide safety and follow the pain*. The counsellor listens for what the client is emotionally touched by (*poignancy*) and makes sure to reflect that back, accurately and with complete unconditional positive regard. Understandably, clients generally start with safer, more peripheral issues and then gradually move towards what is less safe and more central. As they begin counselling, client and counsellor do a kind of dance in which they move bit by bit towards the main therapeutic focus. This is harder than it sounds, because it turns out that you can't just ask the client at the beginning to tell you what the most painful, important bit is. That's because they do not trust you enough yet to feel safe doing so (you have to earn that); it's also the case that they may not yet know, or have the words for it.

So what can you do? First, you can help this process by being completely open and accepting of whatever they have to say. Not being able to accept your client's experience will shut down your empathy, and that will shut down your client.

Second, you can make sure to reflect the more central, difficult bits whenever the client offers them, at a minimum making sure not to deflect the client away from these. A German psychotherapy researcher named Sachse (1990) showed that it's easier for counsellors to deflect clients away from deeper topics than to get them to go deeper. The two segments from Bethany's counselling presented earlier in this chapter illustrate two points in the deepening process: in Segment 4-1 she is talking about her symptoms in general, but in Segment 4-2, 20 minutes later, she is beginning to explore a difficulty in her relationship with her husband.

Third, you can ask the client to be more specific or give examples or more details. In EFC, the pain is often in the details; it's easier for clients to stay away from their painful feelings if they remain at the level of generalities or abstractions. Thus, at the end of Robert's first response in Segment 4-1, he asks Bethany for examples ('And what kinds of things do you think about?').

Fourth, you can use different kinds of empathic exploration responses (as described earlier in this chapter) to give the client opportunities to go deeper. These include empathic formulations ('running a model in your head'), evocative reflections ('like a fuse burning'), empathic conjectures ('also not feeling good enough [about yourself]?').

Fifth, you can use what EFC calls the 'emotion compass' question: What hurts the most here? (See our discussion in Chapter 3 of the core pain stage of the emotional deepening process.) For example, a bit later in the session, Bethany's therapist asks her:

> Robert: Do you have words for the thing about yourself that you are most ashamed of, the thing you are most afraid other people will see about you?

Finally, possibly most important, when your client accesses a painful feeling, it is important to offer empathic affirmations, which offer unconditional caring and warmth, to help the client stay with the painful feeling and more fully appreciate what it is pointing to (see the end of the third counsellor response in Segment 4-2). In this way, client and counsellor can together gradually move, over the course of the early sessions of counselling, towards the client's main therapeutic focus.

Goal and task agreement. Once the client has located their main therapeutic focus, the main thing that feels injured or broken in their life, therapeutic alliance formation moves on to the next stages, in which client and therapist establish a working agreement on what the main goals of therapy are ('goal agreement') and how to get there ('task agreement'). (See Bordin, 1979, for more on this model of therapeutic relationship formation.)

When we talk about *goal agreement* in EFC, we are again not talking about persuading the client to adopt our pre-formed goals for them. The goals have to come from the client, and in general what we are trying to do is to listen for the goals implicit in the client's main difficulties, feed our understanding of these back to the client, adjust our understanding, and offer to work actively with the client on them. Moreover, *task agreement* flows naturally from goal agreement, because EFC includes a rich variety of ways of working towards different client goals. These ways of working are called *tasks* (short for *therapeutic tasks*), which the therapist can offer the client at opportune moments when the client is ready to work on them. In EFC, these moments of opportunity are called *markers*. They are the subject of much of the rest of this book; we provide an overview of EFC tasks in Chapter 5.

Developing a shared case formulation. However, it's usually more complicated than just asking what the client wants to achieve in their counselling and going with whatever task arises from the goal. Instead, we have to direct the focus of our empathic attunement not only to what hurts the most but also towards the client's forward movement. In other words, we help them explore where their sense of personal agency is pointing, what they hope for or want for themselves, or what the things that hurt the most need to heal them. The essential point is that client and counsellor together create a story about how the client's current difficulties came about and what in the client's own internal process and interactions with others maintains them. This story needs to fit the client's experience, make sense or fit together for client and counsellor, and point the way forward in the counselling, identifying not only the goals (what needs to change in order to resolve the main difficulty) but also how to get there (tasks). In EFC, this story is called a *shared case formulation*. Ideally, the words and ideas come from the client and the counsellor just organizes them; but it's OK for the counsellor to make tentative guesses (empathic conjectures), as long as they check with the client and the client is treated as the expert on their case formulation.

EFC case formulations are developed over the course of therapy, gradually emerging from the first session forward. In fact, it can be a tricky, complicated business; Goldman and Greenberg (2014) wrote a whole book on the subject. However, it's best learned a step at a time, with plenty of examples. Here is an extract from the counsellor's process notes for Bethany's first session, focusing largely on the beginnings of this process:

- What is the anxiety breaking in your life?, I asked. C (client): Close friendships; she can't open up enough to develop really deep relationships. I asked how this affects her relationship with her husband; C smiled at the thought of him and her daughter, then told me that he and his family are much more open than she is, sometimes telling her more than she wants to know. She described husband as a '6' on a 7-point openness scale (cf. PQ items), while she is a '2'. I note some vulnerability for her here also, and she almost cries; I offer an empathic conjecture: 'You don't feel worthy of him.' C agrees. C has a deep longing/sadness that wants to get closer to others.
- C says, it's like communion in church, where you don't know just how they do it, but she often holds back from taking part out of uncertainty/fear of doing it wrong.
- What are you afraid people will see about you? I asked: C isn't sure but is aware of a harsh critical voice in her that is always there telling her she isn't worthy. She doesn't know where this comes from. I note her trauma history picked up on the diagnostic interview her researcher did with her before starting therapy, ask if this feels related to her social anxiety.

Initial Narrative Work: Helping the Client Tell Their Story

There is often quite a bit of story-telling in the early sessions of EFC. These stories can be brief (a sentence or two) or extended (taking up much of a session). Counsellors are often impatient with their clients' stories, trying to deflect away from story-telling towards the 'real work' of therapy (talking about emotions, evaluating assumptions, etc.). However, if you simply ignore what the client is saying while waiting for them to finish with the story, you are going to miss out on a lot of important things. As Sarbin (1989) noted, emotions only make sense in the context of stories, and stories are only as interesting as the emotions they involve. Angus and Greenberg (2011) wrote a whole book on working with narrative in EFC. The point is, in EFC the idea is not to stop clients from telling stories (good luck with that!), but rather to help them tell *better* stories: richer, more evocative stories, with telling, poignant details that touch the client, for example, with sadness or anger, or horror or shame. And the emotions don't have to be big, dramatic ones; they can instead deal with unspoken resentments or longings, or fleeting moments of peace, joy or curiosity.

You will know that your client needs to tell you a story when the specific details of a sequence of events come gushing out of them (often not in order), like a garden hose, and it's hard to stop them. In EFC, this is called 'narrative pressure' and it's an indicator ('marker') that the client is ready for you to help them tell their story ('narrative work'). Table 4.2 presents the essentials of this Narrative Retelling task. As an example, in session 2 of Bethany's counselling, she decides she wants to work on an upcoming visit to her parents, who live in another city. She reports that she is worried about conflict with her mother, and then in order to explain her concern she briefly narrates the 'background story' for her present concern, beginning to lay out the difficult history she has had with her mother. Note that the therapist does not sit back and just let the client tell her story, but rather enters imaginatively and actively into the telling, displaying their understanding of each piece of the story as it emerges and filling in possible pieces of the story along the way (narrative elements in italics):

Robert:	So tell me about the worry you have about going to see your parents.
Bethany:	*Well, so like when I was a teenager, my mom and I had difficulties, (T: OK) but it got better since I left the house (T: OK, OK), and I moved out when I was 18.*
Robert:	*Pretty much as soon as you could go.* [empathic reflection]
Bethany:	*I went to Uni, and my mom she still, she has depression, and she has a lot of anxiety, some phobias as well, like going out in crowded places, so she's got a lot going on.*
Robert:	So you can see some of that in you. [empathic conjecture; commentary on narrative]
Bethany:	Yeah, I think some of that is learned.
Robert:	From watching her while you were growing up. [empathic reflection]

Bethany:	Yeah, and so she's like really sensitive, she can see criticisms when there's not criticisms.
Robert:	Right, so you could be complimenting her and she could hear it as a criticism, (C: Yeah) so you have to tread really carefully. [empathic reflection]
Bethany:	(laughs) Yeah and that coupled with the fact that *I* am quite sensitive.
Robert:	(strongly, laughing caringly) You're sensitive too! [empathic affirmation]
Bethany (going back: *to narrative work)*	*Yeah, I think as a teenager growing up, I had to protect myself or just get…*
Robert:	*Rubbed raw emotionally, yeah. [evocative reflection] (C: So …) So you mom could be a bit jagged. In her sensitivity she could say things that actually hurt you in your sensitivity. [empathic formulation of interaction between client and her mother]*
Bethany:	*Yeah, but like when she first got depression, she thought that I was like trying to hurt her and stuff-*
Robert:	*That's right I remember from your intake, that the traumatic event was when your mom got depressed, was it four years or something? [process disclosure of remembered information about client]*
Bethany:	*Yeah it was after my brother was born, and she had post-natal depression. (T: Oh, I see.) That was when I was 14.*
Robert:	Your brother was born, and you saw your mother fall into a hole for 4 years, at least until you left home. [empathic reflection]
Bethany:	*She's still on medication.*
Robert:	*She's never completely recovered from that. [empathic reflection]*
Bethany:	*No she has not.*
Robert:	*Before that, she was…? [exploratory question, encouraging client to go back to an earlier point in the story]*
Bethany:	*She was, I think she still had anxiety stuff, but she had a difficult childhood herself. Her mom had mental health problems.*
Robert:	*So generation after generation, OK. [empathic reflection]*
Bethany:	*So she still had like anxiety issues, because she's kind of deaf as well, she finds it difficult to filter out noise and hear what people are saying.*

Sometimes the client will rush through the story in just a couple of minutes, after which time they will stop and look at you as if to say, 'Now what?'. If the story feels like it is important, that is, if it deals with a painful or traumatic situation or relates to one of the client's main presenting issues (e.g., an unresolved relationship, social anxiety or depression), then you may want to help them go back through the story in greater detail. Three sessions later, in session 5, Bethany came back to this same story as she moved into the middle phase of her counselling (described in Chapters 5–8), working on her harsh internal critic; but the second time she told the story in much greater detail.

Jonah Begins Counselling

In the first session Jonah came in apprehensive about counselling, not knowing what he was getting into. He reported that he wanted to get rid of his depression, was afraid it was getting worse and was interfering with his work and his relationships. He said he had a tendency to not let anybody in, and that he dealt with depression by going to sleep.

His counsellor Margaret, was trained by Les for two years in person-centred counselling, and then for one and a half years in EFC, enabling her to integrate person-centred relational conditions with EFC's marker guided work on tasks. She was supervised by him on this case. Together they watched video recordings of every other session. Margaret started by listening empathically to Jonah's feelings, at first mostly about his depression and anxiety, as they explored his narrative about the problem and gathered information about his early and current relationships. In the first supervision session Margaret and Les discussed Jonah's style of processing emotions, noting that he was somewhat external and tended to talk about his experiences in a third-person manner; however, they also noticed that he occasionally dipped into a more internal focus and showed some emotional arousal, especially when talking about his mother. In the first session, Jonah described how while he was growing up his mother always made him feel like he was doing something terribly wrong. He said he was terrified of being terrified and related this to how, when as a child he was upset, his mother used to say, 'What the hell is the matter with you!' Also, he remembered how as a child he was afraid that if he tried something and failed, it was worse than not trying at all.

Jonah said he feared his emotions and avoided both his anger and his sadness, trying to push them away to keep them under control. He also was embarrassed for feeling anxiety and was always judging himself. In his current life, he said he often felt judged by his wife and felt that he deserved this. The therapist helped him unfold his story and kept a gentle focus on his feelings throughout, while validating how painful it must have been growing up with his mother. At the end of the first session Margaret felt she had made a good connection with Jonah and both she and Les agreed that there appeared to be a clear marker of Unfinished Business (see Chapter 7) with Jonah's mother and that it would be a good idea to see if it continued to emerge in future sessions.

Further Exploration

Reading

Angus, L., & Greenberg, L. S. (2011). *Working with narrative in emotion-focused therapy.* Washington, DC: American Psychological Association.

Elliott, R., Bohart, A. C., Watson, J. C., & Murphy, D. (2018). Therapist empathy and client outcome: An updated meta-analysis. *Psychotherapy, 55,* 399–410. DOI: 10.1037/pst0000175

Elliott, R., Watson, J., Goldman, R. N., & Greenberg, L. S. (2004). *Learning emotion-focused therapy: The process-experiential approach to change.* Washington, DC: American Psychological Association. [See Chapters 7 & 8]

Geller, S. M., & Greenberg, L. S. (2012). *Therapeutic presence: A mindful approach to effective psychotherapy.* Washington, DC: American Psychological Association.

Watching

Elliott, R. (2016). *Developing an Empathic Way of Being with Emotion-Focused Therapy.* Center for Building a Culture of Empathy. Available online at: www.youtube.com/watch?time_continue=2981&v=K4V2yMyv0Po&feature=emb_logo

Reflecting

1. Do the Body Metaphors for Empathy exercise described in Table 4.3. Now reflect on your experience of doing it. Which empathic movement seems to come most naturally for you? Which seems harder, or doesn't quite make sense to you?
2. Pay attention to how present you are when you are around other people. What draws you into stronger connection? What holds you back in being fully present with others? Is it possible to be too present?

5

Early Working Phase: Unfolding and Focusing

Chapter Outline

Overview of Therapeutic Tasks in Emotion-Focused Counselling

Evocative Unfolding of Problematic Reactions

Focusing for an Unclear Feeling

Bethany: Unfolding and Focusing in the Early Working Phase

Further Exploration

Overview of Therapeutic Tasks in Emotion-Focused Counselling

In this and the next three chapters we describe the main therapeutic tasks as they occur in the working ('middle') phase of EFC. In particular we develop the notion of therapeutic tasks, and describe the basics of six key EFC tasks, illustrating these with transcripts from our two case examples. Specifically, in this chapter, we first provide an overview of the nature of markers and tasks, then we move on to working with problematic reactions and unclear feelings. These two tasks often appear early in the working phase of counselling and prepare the way for work on internal conflicts (see Chapter 6) and the tasks of the late working phase of EFC: empty chair work for unresolved relationships (Chapter 7) and empathic affirmation and compassionate self-soothing for painful, vulnerable states (Chapter 8).

As we described in the previous chapter, the general way EFC counsellors work with feelings is through empathic attunement to emotions. This involves *following* clients' emotions, listening moment by moment for what hurts, and helping put those feelings into words (i.e., symbolize them). This main way of relating is then complemented with various types of therapeutic work, sometimes referred to as *experiments*, in which the counsellor offers ways of guiding their client in processing their emotions. To 'experiment' means to try something to see what happens; essentially, the counsellor suggests different ways of working in the session to help the client to access and deepen their emotional experience. One type of experiment involves guiding client attention to attend to their present experience and more specifically to what is going on in their body. Another type of experiment involves re-evoking past experiences to help clients re-live a past moment and is related to the narrative work described in the previous chapter. A third major type of experiment (described in Chapter 6) involves using imagery and psychodrama-type enactments, to explore an internal conflict and to evoke primary feelings. These experiments are referred to as tasks, and are used to help clients explore the specific kinds of concerns they are trying to resolve.

As we have said from the beginning of this book, a defining feature of EFC is that it is *marker guided*. Research has demonstrated that clients bring specific emotional processing difficulties to sessions and that they present these using identifiable *markers*, that is, in-session statements and actions that reveal internal client states of readiness to work on specific immediate emotional difficulties. Thus, they offer opportunities for particular types of therapeutic work or experiment (Greenberg et al., 1993; Rice & Greenberg, 1984). In EFC, client markers are described behaviourally but point to inner client experiences of very particular kinds of emotional difficulty that clients want to work on with the therapist. Emotion-focused counsellors are trained to identify these markers and to offer specific ways to work that best suit these problems. Most of the tasks have been studied both intensively and extensively (Elliott et al., 2004; Greenberg, 2010), so that we now know the key steps towards resolution and what resolution looks like. These models of the actual process of change act as rough maps to guide the counsellor intervention.

The appearance of a marker in the session indicates that the client is trying to resolve a particular type of emotional difficulty. In response, the counsellor attempts to help the client work on the problem, by offering ways of going about it. What is important is that markers indicate that clients are active agents already struggling with trying to solve their own difficulties, with counsellors doing their best to facilitate this process. Tasks are not techniques to modify behaviour but rather are systematic ways of relating with clients that have been found to be helpful for a particular type of processing problem. Thus, these experiments are not engaged in with the intention to fix the client, but rather are offered to clients to help them access, deepen and resolve their emotions. Clients are always seen as experts on their own experience. Clients know what hurts, what is painful and has been pushed away; once they access their emotions with the help of the counsellor, they know what they need and what direction they need to take to heal. Clients are seen as active problem solvers trying to resolve their emotional difficulties. Counsellors, on the other hand, are seen as experts on process facilitation. They offer their expertise in knowing some ways to help clients access and deepen their emotions, and they know something about what kinds of experiments to offer at different moments to facilitate this deepening, with the view that organismic wisdom is embedded in clients' primary emotions.

Table 5.1 provides an overview of the wide range of current EFC markers and their accompanying forms of therapeutic work; these tasks have been identified and are described in detail elsewhere (Elliott et al., 2004; Greenberg et al., 1993; Greenberg & Watson, 2005; Watson & Greenberg, 2017). In this chapter and the next three we provide more detailed descriptions of the most important of these, beginning with (a) *evocative unfolding of problematic reactions*; (b) *focusing for a vague or unclear feeling*; and (c) *two chair dialogue for conflict splits*. These tasks tend to appear earlier in counselling than those in the later chapters, and are characteristic of the early stages of the working phase of EFC as the client begins to grapple with their main issues. In Chapters 7 and 8 we will describe three more key tasks that tend to appear later in the working phase of EFC: (d) empty chair work for unresolved relational issues; (e) empathic affirmation for vulnerability; and (f) compassionate self-soothing for anguish. Several additional tasks are also listed in Table 5.1 and have been described in various sources (see Elliott et al., 2004; Watson & Greenberg, 2017).

TABLE 5.1 *Current EFC tasks*

Marker	Therapeutic Work
A. Interpersonal/Relational Markers:	
1. ***Begins therapy***	Alliance Formation (see Chapter 4)
2. ***Alliance Difficulty***: (a) Confrontation: Expresses or implies complaint or dissatisfaction about nature or progress of therapy, or therapeutic relationship; (b) Withdrawal: disengages from therapy process.	Relational Dialogue
3. ***Vulnerability***: Expresses distress over present strong negative self-related feelings (usually with hopelessness and sense of isolation).	Empathic Affirmation *(alternate: Compassionate Self-soothing)* (Chapter 8)
4. ***Contact Disturbance***: Immediate in-session state takes client out of psychological contact with therapist (hearing voices, dissociation, panic, narrowly focused interest).	Contact Work (Pre-therapy)
B. Experiencing Markers:	
1. ***Unclear Feeling***: (a) Vague/nagging concern; (b) global, abstract, superficial, or externalized mode of engagement.	Focusing (Chapter 5)
2. ***Attentional Focus Difficulty***: (a) Overwhelmed by multiple worries or one big worry; (b) stuck/blank: unable to find a session focus.	Clearing a Space (See Reflection Activity 4 at end of this chapter)
C. Reprocessing Markers:	
1. ***Narrative pressure***: Refers to a traumatic/painful experience about which a story wants to be told (e.g., traumatic event, disrupted life story, nightmare).	Narrative Retelling *(can be enacted with chairs)* (Chapter 4)

(Continued)

TABLE 5.1   *(Continued)*

Marker	Therapeutic Work
2. **Problematic Reaction Point**: Describes unexpected, puzzling personal reaction (behaviour, emotion reaction).	Evocative Unfolding *(can be enacted)* (Chapter 5)
3. **Meaning Protest**: Describes a life event discrepant with cherished beliefs, in an emotionally aroused state.	Meaning Re-Creation
D. Configuration/Introject Markers:	
1. **Conflict Split**: Describes conflict between two aspects of self, in which one aspect of self is (a) critical (self-criticism split), (b) coercive towards (coaching and motivational splits), or (c) blocks another aspect (self-interruption split).	Two Chair Dialogue (with two self-aspects) *(Alternate: Configuration Work)* (Chapter 6)
2. **Attribution Split**: Describes overreaction to others, in which others are experienced as (a) critical of, (b) coercive towards, or (c) blocking of the self.	Two Chair Work (with Others as one self-aspect) *(Alternate: Configuration Work re: imagined Others)* (Chapter 6)
3. **Unresolved Relationship Issues (Unfinished Business)**: Blames, complains or expresses hurt or longing in relation to a significant other.	Empty Chair Work *(Alternate: Speaking Your Truth Work)* (Chapter 7)
4. **Anguish**: Expresses strong emotional pain primarily based on old, familiar experiences of severe self-criticism or lack of connection/support.	Compassionate Self-soothing *(Alternate: Empathic Affirmation)* (Chapter 8)

Evocative Unfolding of Problematic Reactions

One of the first EFC tasks to be identified was *evocative unfolding for problematic reaction points* (Rice & Saperia, 1984), a rather difficult piece of EFC jargon that needs to be unpacked. Let's start with 'problematic reaction points'. Clients signal that they are ready to work on this task when they tell us they are puzzled by how they felt or what they did in a particular situation. For instance, one client said, 'It's so strange: on the way to therapy today I saw a little puppy dog with long droopy ears and I suddenly felt so sad. I don't know why I reacted like that.' Here, 'problematic' means puzzling or not understood; 'reaction' means something the client (not someone else) personally felt or did; and 'point' refers to a specific moment (point in time) rather than a general tendency or pattern. Examples we see often in counselling are anger or anxiety episodes, eating or substance misuse difficulties, and puzzling interpersonal activities such as affairs.

Next, let's look at the 'evocative unfolding' part. Problematic reactions are opportunities for the counsellor to offer the client the chance to evoke – vividly re-experience – the situation and their emotional reaction to it by 'unfolding' it, that is, by going back over it slowly and carefully. The idea is to re-establish the connection between the situation and the client's reaction. The point is to arrive at the implicit meaning of the situation that makes sense of the puzzling reaction; when this happens, the client comes to understand their reaction and no longer feels puzzled by it. However, understanding my reaction then opens up a larger question: What is it about my general ways of processing my emotions that leads me to react in this way? Fuller resolution involves considering new ways of seeing self and others and an exploration of the contrast between old versus new views and the emotions that go along with these.

Table 5.2 lays out the sequence of steps in exploring these problematic reactions. First, the counsellor identifies the reaction that the client feels is puzzling in some way and proposes the task. Second, the counsellor asks the client to provide a vivid description of the scene in which the client was a participant when their reaction occurred. Together, client and counsellor evoke and recapture a graphic sense of the situation ('scene building'), with the therapist using exploratory questions and evocative reflections. Third, once the scene has been vividly recreated, the counsellor directs the client to search for the particularly salient (emotionally powerful) aspects of the situation that triggered the reaction. Fourth, after clients identify what was salient about the situation, they are able to determine how they construed (made sense of) the stimulus so as to arrive at an understanding of its personal meaning for them. This *meaning bridge* helps clients understand their reaction better. Fifth, the counsellor may then support the client in exploring the emotion scheme (see Chapter 2) that was activated by the problematic situation. The client becomes aware of their personal style or general way of responding so that they can then examine it to understand its origins and determine whether it is still useful; this often reveals a conflict between old and new ways of experiencing situations, leading to two chair work (described in Chapter 6). Sixth, following the exploration of the emotion scheme the client is able to come up with alternative ways of responding or of construing the situation. The aim of using systematic evocative unfolding is to have clients re-experience as fully as possible the problematic situation so that they can symbolize it more accurately in awareness and then discover the personal impact or meaning of the situation; this helps them access new emotion schemes, with alternative needs and action tendencies (Rice & Saperia, 1984).

TABLE 5.2 *Evocative unfolding for problematic reactions: Task resolution model*

Client Resolution Stage	Counsellor Facilitating Responses
1. *Marker confirmation*: Client describes unexpected, puzzling personal reaction.	• Identify and reflect marker to client to make sure you understand it. • Propose task and see if client wants to do it.
2. *Re-evoking experience*: Client re-enters scene and recalls and re-experiences specific moment when reaction was triggered.	• Encourage client to re-enter and re-experience the situation in their mind's eye ('scene building').
3. *Tracking the two sides*: Client recalls salient aspects of stimulus situation and explores their internal emotional reactions to the situation and the sense or meaning (subjective construal) they made of it.	• Help client explore their perception of external situation, their internal reaction, and the connection between these. • Help client to redirect attention between external situation and internal reaction, as needed to keep the work moving forward.

(Continued)

TABLE 5.2 *(Continued)*

Client Resolution Stage	Counsellor Facilitating Responses
4. *Meaning bridge (partial resolution)*: Client discovers the connection between their puzzling reaction and how they perceived the situation.	• Listen for and reflect possible meaning bridges. • Assess client's continuing sense of being puzzled to see if resolution has occurred. • Use empathic conjecture to offer possible meaning bridges. • Help client to frame the broader issue.
5. *Recognizing and re-examining self-related emotion schemes*: Client recognizes reaction as an example of a broader habitual mode of seeing self and others; explores alternate self-related emotion schemes and their consequences.	• Listen for and help client to explore broader meanings and implications that emerge. • Help client to explore alternate self-schemes and possible conflict between these. • Offer two chair work as appropriate to facilitate this (see Chapter 6).
6. *Considering new options (full resolution)*: Client gains new view of important aspects of own functioning and desired self-change; begins to feel empowered to make changes.	• Listen for and explore emerging new self-understandings and implications for change.

A brief example of the process of resolving a problematic reaction with Jonah, our depressed male client, helps us see how the client came to a new awareness of himself and the problem that he needed to work on in therapy. (The example is brief, highlighting key examples of work at each stage; work on this task typically takes much of a counselling session.) The client started out by describing his reaction:

Jonah:	I had a fight with my wife this morning before I left for my office and I've just been feeling so bummed out all day. I just don't know why it got to me so much that it affected me all day.
Margaret:	What happened this morning?
Jonah:	Well I was getting ready to leave and then she shouted down to me to not forget to get the car in for repairs and to make sure I got home in time as we were going out tonight.

Together, client and counsellor then worked to rebuild and recapture a vivid sense of the situation:

Margaret:	So where were you when this happened? [Scene building exploratory question]
Jonah:	I was standing at the bottom of the stairs ready to leave for work and she had just got up and was at the top yelling down to me.
Margaret:	So there you were, suit and tie, briefcase in your hand, your wife at the top in her dressing gown shouting down to you. [Evocative reflection]

Next, once the scene had been vividly recreated by the participants, the counsellor directed Jonah to attend to his bodily felt reaction:

Margaret: So you just maybe felt this tightening up in your body? [Empathic conjecture]
Jonah: Well, no, actually I felt this kind of sinking feeling in my stomach.

They also searched for the particularly salient aspect of the situation that triggered the reaction:

Margaret: I see, just a sinking feeling, and somehow, something you heard, saw or sensed triggered this… [Exploratory reflection]
Jonah: Well, I could just see her standing up there. Something about her expression.
Margaret: I see. Her face, something about her expression.
Jonah: Yeah, she just was so contemptuous in her face and voice.
Margaret: Contempt… Looking down on you. [Evocative reflection]

After Jonah identified what was salient about the situation, he was able to determine how he construed or made sense of the stimulus, which enabled him to arrive at an understanding of its personal meaning:

Jonah: It was like belittling, like she was saying, 'I know you'll forget, you'll screw it up, something won't work'. Yeah, it was the contempt and this so reminds me of my mother. She never thought I did anything right. It was like, 'Do it, but I know you will screw up.'

This meaning bridge helped Jonah to understand his reaction better. Then he began to elaborate the emotion scheme that was activated by the problematic situation. Jonah became aware of his personal reaction to his wife. The counsellor then went on to help the client unpack his construal of the situation to try to understand how he interpreted it so as to understand its idiosyncratic meaning for the client and its relevance to the way he was operating in the world. By carefully and slowly focusing the client on his reaction and his construal of events the counsellor was thus able to help him identify what triggered him and get to its origins that affected his style of being in the world: always feeling inadequate and expecting criticism from important others. In later sessions they reprocessed Jonah's unresolved issues with his mother using an empty chair dialogue (see Chapter 7).

Practising the evocative unfolding task helps counsellors learn how to work with *episodic memories*, that is, memories for specific things that have happened, helping clients to learn to use these memories to bring them to life and access specific emotions more strongly. Episodic memories are important in other tasks, especially the different forms of chair work covered in Chapters 6 and 7.

Focusing for an Unclear Feeling

Another key task in EFC is *focusing for an unclear feeling*. As noted in Chapter 1, focusing is a body of person-centred-experiential counselling practice originally developed by

Gendlin (1981) and others (e.g., Cornell, 1996). Its six-step formulation made it quite easy to adapt into EFC practice. In addition, from an EFC point of view, its key idea, referred to as the *felt sense* by Gendlin and others, corresponds closely to what EFC calls an *emotion scheme*.

In EFC terms, the marker for focusing is an *unclear feeling*, in which the person is confused about what they feel, or finds they are talking around in a circle on the surface of their experience: 'I just have this feeling but I don't know what it is.' An unclear feeling calls for *focusing* (Cornell, 1996; Gendlin, 1981), in which the counsellor invites the client to approach the bodily aspects of their unclear feeling with attention, patience, and curiosity, in order to experience it more fully and to find words or images that will accurately symbolize it. Resolution involves a *felt shift* in the person's body (usually a release of tension), creation of new meaning, and a sense of forward movement in the person's life. In addition, bits of focusing are used in a range of other tasks, especially two chair and empty chair work.

In *focusing*, the counsellor guides the client through a series of steps, outlined in Table 5.3.

TABLE 5.3   *Focusing for unclear feelings: Task resolution model*

Client Resolution Stage	Counsellor Facilitating Responses
1. *Marker: Unclear Feeling*: Rich, complex or troubling sense of something (also: vague, stuck, blank, global, external).	• Identify, reflect marker to client; propose task; or ask client to identity *something* to attend to. • Suggest client take a deep breath, set aside other issues for now.
2. *Attending* to the unclear feeling, including their whole sense of it.	Encourage *focusing attitude*: • Invite client to turn compassionate attention inward to unclear or troubling bodily feelings. • What feelings in my body? Where? • Encourage attitude of receptive waiting. • Encourage attention to *whole* feeling. • What is this about? What gets it so _____?
3. *Symbolizing and checking* potential descriptions: Client develops label, symbolic representation; also checks accuracy of label.	• Ask client to find word or image for unclear feeling. • Reflect exactly what client says; avoid interpretation. • Encourage client to compare label to unclear feeling, until 'fit' is found.
4. *Asking*: Client either experiences relief from accurately labelling the feeling; or if stuck, asks further questions of the feeling.	Use exploratory shift questions: • What is most difficult or painful about it? • What does it want/need?
5. *Receiving the feeling shift*: Appreciating, consolidating feeling shift.	• Encourage client to stay with feeling that has shifted. • Help client to temporarily set aside critical or opposing feelings.
6. *Carrying forward* outside therapy; or new in-session task.	Listen for, facilitate carrying forward if appropriate (what is next? where does it lead?)

The first step is the marker: a description of some kind of unclear feeling, as in this idealized example,

Darius (client):	So, I'm having these feelings about my relationship right now, but it's really hard to describe them. It's kind of like irritation or crankiness, but that isn't quite right either. It's really hard to say what they are but they don't feel good....

Typically, the counsellor then next offers the focusing task by asking the client if they can turn their attention inward to the throat/chest/stomach area of their body; this is the *attending* stage of focusing. You are looking for a description of a physical sensation, such as tightness, a knot, emptiness or heaviness, or pain:

Keisha (counsellor):	It involves kind of looking inside yourself, making a bit of space inside yourself. Maybe take a breath and see if you can get comfortable. (Pause.) Now try asking yourself: What am I feeling right now in my body? What is there for me? Take a minute to try that. (Pause.) Let me know what comes to you. (Pause.)
Darius:	It feels, erh, tight.

The counsellor might then ask the client to say where in their body they feel the tightness, to which the client might say:

Darius:	It's in my diaphragm area.

After reflecting this, the counsellor might ask the client to gently put a hand where the feeling is happening in their body.

It is important to ask your client if it is OK to pay attention to this feeling, because it might be uncomfortable or overwhelming:

Keisha:	Is it OK to stay with this right now even though it might be scary?

The counsellor can help the client accept and stay with their feeling by suggesting that they be caring and interested in their sense even though it is unclear or uncomfortable, trying to accept it as an important part of them that is trying to tell them something. Then they might ask the client what in their relation gets their body to feel so tight:

Darius:	I feel like I'm failing him; I'm always working, and don't give him enough attention, and he's really unhappy.

After reflecting this, the counsellor then typically guides the client through the third stage, which is a process of *symbolizing and checking* back and forth between the feeling and the potential labels for it to find the one that fits best:

Keisha:	Take a minute and see if you can find a word or image that captures the whole quality of this feeling, you know, like a metaphor or something that symbolizes the whole thing.
Darius:	(Pause) Umm… it's kinda like a jagged rock, like a chunk of granite, all sharp edges.
Keisha:	A sharp, jagged piece of granite, right there in your chest… Does that fit the feeling with your partner? Ask yourself and see.
Darius:	No, not exactly, it's more alive, it feels more like a crab, with hard, sharp claws, and it won't let go.
Keisha:	Does that fit? A kind of clutching crab and it's sharp and I guess it hurts.
Darius:	Yes.

Sometimes, all it takes for a *feeling shift* (Stage 5) to occur is for the unclear feeling to be clearly symbolized. At other times, however, even though the feeling has been clarified, it does not shift, generally because it is an old stuck bad feeling (primary maladaptive emotion). In this case, the counsellor helps the client to deepen the stuck emotion by asking exploratory questions (Stage 4: *Asking*):

Keisha:	I hear that. And maybe you could ask it, what is most difficult or painful about this clutching crab feeling?
Darius:	That the sharp, jaggedness of the crab will drive everyone away and the pain will never end.
Keisha:	Wow! That there will be nobody there and you'll always feel so alone, that feels almost unbearable?
Darius:	Yes.
Keisha:	And what does that pain and loneliness need?
Darius:	Just someone who isn't scared of it and who won't abandon me.
Keisha:	Just someone to stay by you and see past the sharp claws to the part of you that's so scared and lonely and vulnerable.
Darius:	(sighing, letting his breath out) Yes (crying). Yes…

In this last response, the sighing and tears indicate that the feeling has changed from maladaptive to adaptive, marking the beginning of the fifth stage, *receiving the feeling shift*. Here the counsellor encourages the client to stay with the new feeling and the relief that comes with it, in order to appreciate it and to set aside any secondary critical reactions to the shift.

The final, optional stage, is *carrying forward*, in which the client might continue experiential work in session with the therapist or alternatively might want to consider the potential implications of the feeling shift for their life outside counselling:

Keisha:	So where does this leave you? What do you want to do with it, if anything?
Darius:	I'm not sure, I guess right now it feels tender and special. I just want to take the sad feeling away with me and maybe give it some space and be gentle with it.

This step also involves making sure that the client is OK with where they have ended, especially if the client has more work to do on the issue.

Although it is not used extensively by itself, EFC counsellors make frequent use of aspects of the focusing process. These include the use of open, exploratory questions about immediate experience; encouraging clients to put their hand on the bodily feeling while the counsellor nonverbally mirrors the gesture; the use of *fit questions* about whether a potential description of a feeling fits the feeling or not; paying attention to bodily shifts and encouraging clients to stay with these when they occur; and so on. For this reason, learning the focusing task will strengthen your EFC practice in general and is well worth the effort.

Bethany: Unfolding and Focusing in the Early Working Phase

Bethany's session 3 is the beginning of the working phase of her counselling and includes both tasks described in this chapter. Bethany comes into the session feeling anxious from travelling on a crowded bus to get there, but also worried that she doesn't know what to talk about (a key feature of her social anxiety). The therapist guides her through a few minutes of evocative unfolding of the bus journey, as an example of her fear of other people, and helps her describe how her internal conversation went as she was sitting on the bus. She reports telling herself that she might choose a topic she thinks is safe but that turns out not to be safe, and then she might feel trapped. Bethany goes on to say that she's also afraid of running out of things to say, resulting in awkward silences in the session; she is also afraid of wasting the therapist's time, and fears that the therapist might be annoyed at her for wasting his time. Looking upset, she admits that she would also be annoyed at herself for wasting time. This worry makes it difficult for her to talk to other people and was a lot of what was bothering her on her journey to the session.

Client and counsellor go on exploring Bethany's experiences of social situations more generally, then she moves into a story about a crisis in her marriage when her husband challenged her to open up to him. After she finishes the story, there is an awkward pause. At this point, the counsellor proposes that they do a bit of focusing: 'Can you take a minute and ask yourself, "What am I experiencing right now?"' Bethany says that she's not as anxious as earlier, but that there is still a tight knot in her chest. The counsellor asks her to focus on this knot in her chest, suggesting that she try to remember what she felt during the awkward pause. He asks her what the tight knot is about. After looking inside, Bethany describes it as being brought on by her internal guarding and self-critical voices. After processing this work for a bit, client and therapist move on to two chair work, which is the subject of Chapter 6.

Further Exploration

Reading

Cornell, A. W. (1996). *The power of focusing*. Oakland, CA: New Harbinger.
Elliott, R., Watson, J. C., Goldman, R. N., & Greenberg, L. S. (2004). *Learning emotion-focused therapy: The process-experiential approach to change*. Washington, DC: American Psychological Association. [See Chapter 11]

Watson, J. C., & Rennie, D. (1994). A qualitative analysis of clients' reports of their subjective experience while exploring problematic reactions in therapy. *Journal of Counseling Psychology, 41*, 500–509.

Watching

Elliott, R. (2018). *Resolving Problematic Reactions in Emotion-Focused Therapy*. American Psychological Association Videos. [Demonstration of systematic evocative unfolding]
Greenberg, L. S. (2007). *Emotion-Focused Therapy over Time (Psychotherapy in Six Sessions)*. [Video]. Washington, DC: American Psychological Association (Producer). [See beginning of session 2]

Reflecting

1. Take a look back at Table 5.1. Which of the EFC tasks described there would you like to learn more about? Which ones don't appeal to you? Why?
2. Using your own experience, think of a recent example of an *unclear feeling*, where you had a general or vague sense of something that was bothering you that you had trouble putting into words. Write a brief description of this experience.
3. See if you can think of an example of a *problematic reaction point* that you have experienced, in which you found yourself feeling or doing something that left you feeling puzzled about why you reacted in that way. Write a brief description of this experience.
4. Are you feeling overwhelmed by too many demands or worries? If so, try this variation of the Focusing task, called *Clearing a Space* (Elliott et al., 2004):
   a. Take a breath, get comfortable and try to slow yourself down.
   b. Ask yourself, 'What is one thing that's keeping me from feeling good right now?' Be patient, and let it come to you.
   c. When a concern comes to you, imagine setting it aside, either in the room or space you are in right now, or in a favourite space or place. If you need to, imagine putting the concern in a box or other container. Pay attention to what happens.
   d. Repeat this process until you run out of concerns to set aside.
   e. Sit with the feeling of having all these concerns set aside; let yourself feel what this feels like.

6

Early Working Phase: Two Chair Work

Chapter Outline

Overview of Two Chair Dialogue for Internal Conflicts

Predialogue and Entry Stages

Deepening and Emerging Shift Stages

Softening/Negotiation and Postdialogue Stages

Working with Other Kinds of Conflicts

Bethany: Two Chair Work in the Early Working Phase

Further Exploration

Overview of Two Chair Dialogue for Internal Conflicts

In this chapter we provide an overview of how to work with *conflict split* markers and the two chair dialogue task. This task is often the first psychodramatic experiment used and usually takes place early in the working phase of counselling. In this task the counsellor guides the client to 'experiment' with having a dialogue between two parts of the self. The task involves using imagery and enactments, to explore an internal conflict between two parts of the self and to evoke primary feelings. Often one voice or part is critical of another part of the self.

The conflict split marker. In the conflict split task marker, one aspect of the self treats another aspect negatively, being critical, coercive or interruptive towards it. For example, a woman might quickly become both hopeless and defeated but also angry in the face of failure in the eyes of her sisters:

Client: I feel inferior to them. It's like 'I've failed and I'm not as good as them.'

As Table 6.1 indicates, there are many types of conflict split; it is the most common and varied of all EFC task markers. However, three are fundamental to all the others, based on the different types of negative treatment of self (see the first three rows in Table 6.1). The most common and basic of all these is the *self-critical split*, such as the one above, in which one part of the self attacks another part. Self-critical splits involve some form of *self-evaluation*: 'I feel inferior', 'I've failed and I'm worthless', or 'I am not a good enough mother/wife/friend/worker, etc.'. We refer to one side as the *critic* and the other as the *experiencing self* or *experiencer*. This kind of conflict is often between internalized self-critical evaluations on one side and organismic feelings and associated needs and wants on the other. *Self-coercion splits* involve a controlling part of us putting pressure on another part, for example, to work harder, to go the gym when we don't feel like it, or more generally to be perfect. Finally, in *self-interruption splits* we try to block our-selves from saying, doing or even feeling something, for example, we silence ourselves, paralyze ourselves, or shut down our anger or emotional pain. Both self-coercion and self-interruption involve attempts to control ourselves that readily take on elements of self-criticism when the other part does not comply.

As can be seen in Table 6.1, there are also many more specific kinds of conflict; however, they all derive from the three fundamental kinds of negative treatment of self. For example, in *attribution splits* we attribute or project one aspect of self onto others, usually the part that is doing the negative treatment of self. Thus, we may be afraid of other people judging us when it is really our internal critic that we are projecting onto them. In *anxiety splits*, one part is a catastrophizer and the other part is the anxious experience: the catastrophizer is a combination of a controlling part and a critic that is trying to keep the person safe from bad things happening, but does this by regularly scaring the anxious part, so that they end up feeling even less safe. *Self-coaching* splits can be confusing because they are second-level criticisms that mask an underlying criticism. They arise when people are criticizing them-selves for having a problem like being depressed or procrastinating when the real underly-ing process is criticizing or making themselves anxious for character flaws. Underneath 'You are bad for being depressed' the underlying criticism is 'You are worthless/stupid/ etc.'. Therefore, it's better to help the client move beyond the surface split ('You are bad for having the problem') and work instead on the self-criticism that generates the problem.

TABLE 6.1   *Examples of conflict split marker*

Name	Negative Treatment of Self	Example
Self-criticism	Attack, blame, put down	'That was a stupid thing to say.'
Self-coercion	Force, push, pressurize	'You have to be perfect.'
Self-interruption	Block, prevent, stop, silence	'You can't say/do/feel that.'
Attribution	Imagine others treating self negatively	'Everyone thinks you are stupid/have to be perfect/shouldn't do that.'

Name	Negative Treatment of Self	Example
Decisional	Hesitate/vacillate/be torn	'I can't decide whether to stay in this relation/job/city or leave.'
Depressive	Depress yourself	'You're a failure and there is no hope for you.'
Anxiety	Make yourself anxious	'You'd better be careful; you're going to screw this up again.'
Motivational/ Self-damaging	Fail to take care of yourself	'I worry about my drinking, but I'm getting better/it's not so bad/other people are worse.'
Coaching (second-level self-criticism)	Criticize, blame for having a problem	'You are bad for being so depressed, procrastinating.'
Toxic/ Destructive	Destroy yourself	'You don't deserve to live; you should never have been born.'

Two chair dialogue. These markers offer opportunities for *two chair work*: two parts of the self are put into live contact with each other. Thoughts, feelings, and needs within each part of the self are separated out, usually into two chairs, so that they can be explored and communicate with one another directly in a dialogue to achieve a softening of the critical, coercive or interrupting voice. Resolution involves a softening of the negative treatment of self and an integration between the sides. We will focus here primarily on self–critical splits, using them as a prototype for the task in general. Table 6.2 summarizes the stages of two chair dialogue.

TABLE 6.2 *Two chair dialogue for conflict splits: Task resolution model*

Task Resolution Stage	Therapist Responses
1. *Predialogue*:	
1a. *Establishing task collaboration*	• Identify client marker
1b. *Marker expression and agreement*: Expresses negative treatment of self (critical, coercive, interruptive)	• Establish client task collaboration • Structure (set up) experiment
2. *Entering*:	
2a. *Identifying and separating* two aspects of self (negative treatment of self and reaction)	• Create separation and contact between the two aspects
2b. Aspects begin to *interact directly and take responsibility* in a concrete, specific manner	• Promote taking responsibility for each aspect's position • Intensify client arousal

(Continued)

TABLE 6.2   *(Continued)*

Task Resolution Stage	Therapist Responses

3. *Deepening*:
   3a. *Accessing/heightening negative treatment* of self
   3b. *Deepening in the Experiencer*
   3c. *Specifying core negative treatment of self* (defects, injunctions)
   3d. *Continuing to access/express underlying feelings* in the Experiencer and Critic
	• Promote awareness of negative treatment of self (self-criticisms/injunctions/interruptions)
	• Access/express/differentiate underlying feelings/organismic needs in the experiencing aspect
	• Follow deepening forms of the conflict
	• *With collapsed Experiencer: accept/deepen/differentiate hopelessness; or encourage greater specificity in Critic*

4. *Emerging shift: Primary underlying feelings/needs emerge* and are clearly expressed by Experiencer	Facilitate emergence of new organismic feelings: • Help client to stay with and accept their core pain • Differentiate quality of the core pain • Gently inquire about feelings and needs

5. *Softening and negotiation*:
   5a. Negative treatment aspect accesses and expresses *inner experience* and differentiates *values and standards*
   5b. Both aspects show *compassion/concern/respect* for each other
   5c. Clear understanding of how aspects/feelings/needs/wishes may be accommodated/reconciled
   5d. Alternatively: Reject destructive introjected negative aspect
	• Facilitate softening in Critic (into empathy or compassion)
	• Differentiate values and standards in the critical aspect
	• Facilitate mutual understanding/acceptance between aspects
	• Facilitate back-and-forth negotiation between aspects of self: practical compromises
	• *Alternatively: reject destructive introjected voice*

6. *Postdialogue creation of meaning* (with or without resolution): Comes to a better understanding of how their process works and how to move forward	• Collaborate with client to help them to reflect on the work in order to create a shared meaning perspective/formulation • Offer awareness homework (where appropriate)

In brief, when a self-critical marker appears in the client's presentation, the counsellor asks the client to engage in a dialogue between the critical part and the experiencing part of the self (Greenberg, 1984a; Greenberg et al., 1993). In this dialogue, the critical voice and the voice of the experiencing self are first separated and then put into direct contact with each other in a psychodramatic enactment (Greenberg et al., 1993). An important first step is for the counsellor to help the client separate out the voices of the inner critic and self-experiencer; the self-criticisms of the critic are expressed to the experiencer and are differentiated to get to a core self-criticism, such as 'You could have been a somebody, and look at you now; you are a nobody'. If you miss this step, the chair work is likely to feel messy and confusing. Next, the primary painful feelings and needs of the experiencing self, such as sadness or shame, are explored and expressed in the dialogue until the relationship between the voices evolves from one of conflict and blame to one of listening. Resolution then occurs by a softening of the critical voice, often into compassion or empathy, after which negotiation and integration of the sides becomes possible, resulting in the person feeling whole again and no longer split. The steps in the two chair process are described below following a six-stage resolution model (Table 6.2), with examples from Jonah's fourth session.

Many counsellors approaching EFC for the first time may be uncomfortable with all of this talk of furniture and psychodramatic enactments. It can sound quite directive, and indeed when not done properly clients can feel misunderstood, controlled or even threatened or scared. The fact is, chair work simply won't work in the absence of a strong, genuine, caring, empathic counselling relationship. It should not be offered before session 3 or 4, and should never be imposed on unwilling clients. It is most effective when it is a truly collaborative process in which a counsellor is working alongside a client who controls the work. We will try to show you what this looks like with our two running case examples.

Predialogue and Entry Stages

Stage 1. Predialogue. In the predialogue stage, the counsellor identifies the split and empathically reflects the two sides of the self-critical process:

> *Margaret:*   So it's like there is this painful struggle inside: One part is chastising you, saying something like, 'You're not good enough, you never get things right', and another part that feels like, 'I've failed', and feels sort of almost hopeless. Does that sort of capture it?

The first step involves *establishing collaboration and allowing marker expression and agreement*. Once a split marker has been identified and empathized with, the counsellor enlists the client's agreement to work on the split. The counsellor provides a rationale for how engaging in chair work might be helpful, such as:

> *Margaret:*   It helps to bring these voices out into the open so we can see them, or work with them more directly.

The client then says:

> *Jonah:*   I always end up putting myself down like I didn't do a good enough job.
> *Margaret:*   Let's try something? This may sound strange, but sometimes it really does help if we can kind of get those criticisms out in the open, OK? (Jonah: OK). So I'm going to suggest we have a dialogue between your critical voice and yourself. Are you OK with trying this? (Jonah: OK)

	OK, let's have you sit over here, [Jonah moves to critic chair] and this is the side that criticizes you. What do you say to him? [Margaret points to experiencer chair] It's something like, 'You failed, you haven't gotten anywhere?' I don't know the exact messages. Can you articulate some of them, and say them to yourself sitting here.
Jonah:	Uhm Uhhuh. OK.
Margaret:	This part is a kind of critic, an evaluator right? So criticize yourself.
Jonah:	And talk to the chair, don't look at you?
Margaret:	Yeah. Just criticize yourself. Let's get at the messages that you give yourself. How do you criticize yourself, how do you put yourself down?

Stage 2a. Entering: Identifying and separating the aspects. Having established agreement to work using two chair dialogue, the counsellor helps the client with *identifying and separating* the two opposing aspects, as clearly as possible, and works to fully develop each side of the dialogue. Once the critical voice is activated, the counsellor asks the client to move to the self-chair and asks, 'And what do you feel inside when you hear that?' Often the experiencer agrees with the critic or defends against the criticism. These are secondary reactive emotions and ultimately will not be productive processes, so it is important not to dwell on them or promote them. Instead, the counsellor guides the client to focus on what is felt in the body in the present. It is important for the counsellor to be clear that this dialogue is not about whether the criticism is true or not, but about what it feels like to be criticized. The purpose of the dialogue is to access emotion; emotion is based on what is good for me or bad for me, not on what is rational or true or false.

After a few minutes of developing the critic, and ideally when the negative attitude of contempt of the critic has been identified and expressed, and possibly some specific instances exemplifying this criticism, the counsellor suggests that the client move to the experiencer chair to experience what it feels like to be criticized in this way. EFC uses the Focusing process to do this (see Chapter 4). The self is asked what it feels in its body, in response to the criticisms. It is important to get the self's differentiated emotional reaction to the critic and not just a global reaction, such as 'I feel bad'. Instead, the client is guided to pay attention inwards and to get a more differentiated sense that has been activated in the body in the moment. The bodily feeling and action tendency need to be symbolized. The next step in Jonah's dialogue follows:

Margaret:	OK, can you come over here. [Jonah switches chairs.] This is the feeling side, what do you feel right now in your body in response to that?
Jonah [as Experiencer]:	I don't know, but mostly I mean I just feel useless in a way. I sort of agree (laughs).
Margaret:	Yeah, but how do these criticisms make you feel? How do you feel in your body, maybe in your chest or your arms? Anything there?
Jonah:	Well I sort of feel tense, tight in my chest, like I can't breathe.
Margaret:	Tell him.

Jonah:	I feel tense and tight and I sort of collapse. I'll never be able to be strong enough confident enough to assert myself and stand up to my boss or anyone.
Margaret:	Yeah, so just a feeling of collapsing. Will you come over here and let's see what happens inside to make him collapse. [Jonah switches chairs.] What is it you say to yourself?
Jonah [as Critic]:	You, you're weak.
Margaret:	Oh, so you're weak? Say some more.
Jonah:	Yeah. You're spineless, you can't stand up for yourself. If you say something, you'll probably screw it up. Whatever you say, it won't make a difference.
Margaret:	Can you be specific? Like when, tell him when he didn't stand up for himself.
Jonah:	Like yesterday when your boss laid that extra work on you, you just took it without saying you already had your hands full.

Stage 2b. Entering: Interacting directly and taking responsibility. The counsellor now helps the client maintain separation while the client *contacts* and *takes responsibility* for each of the two sides, thus promoting each side's position. This is done by continuously ensuring that the client speaks from the chair in which they are situated. The one voice is critical, the other voice is the experience of being criticized. This is helped by encouraging the client to use 'You' statements when speaking from the critical chair, to capture the blaming quality of this side, and 'I' statements when speaking from the Experiencer, to capture feelings. Each side needs to own its position and to express itself, rather than talk about the other part's experience.

As we saw above when the response at stage 2 from the Experiencing self to the Critic is one of agreement ('You're right'), this agreement should not be taken as face value, because then the split can be lost. Instead, the underlying feeling behind the agreement needs to be focused on and explored or sometimes reflected briefly and then bypassed, in order to get to more fundamental aspects of the self-criticism. The process the counsellor needs to get to in the exploration is that between the critical stance that is involved in creating the depression, such as 'You're worthless', and the initial depressed response of the experiencing self of 'I feel hopeless'.

Deepening and Emerging Shift Stages

This is the stage in which deeper feelings of the self are accessed. One of the main purposes of activating the critical voice in the beginning is to bring alive the person's feeling of what it's like to experience the criticism. At first, it may be more of a secondary feeling like hopelessness or even an angry reaction. Once the client reacts from their experience, the counsellor guides them to attend to their bodily felt experience and attend not only to their first reactions but to what else they may feel. Often self-criticism activates core feelings of worthlessness, inadequacy, and shame. In this part of the dialogue the client goes back and forth a few times to get to core criticisms and needs to get very specific and concrete in explicating what they say to themselves. This helps deepen the client's painful emotions when responding from the experiencer chair. Once the emotion has been deepened and the painful feelings accessed, the associated unmet needs will emerge and a sense of deserving to have the need met often helps the client to shift to a stronger sense of self-worth.

Stage 3a. Deepening: Accessing and heightening negative treatment of self. Continuing with Jonah's dialogue below, he is now in the Experiencing chair and is responding to the critical voice's statement that he is a failure. We can see here in the Experiencing chair how he begins to differentiate his bad feelings into 'nervous' and 'dread that something bad will happen'. The dialogue then shifts to more of anxiety-creating dialogue ('anxiety split'), in which the critic acts more as a catastrophizing, controlling voice:

Margaret:	What happens for you here?
Jonah [as Experiencer]:	Well, I get nervous, I don't know, I get a feeling inside… afraid that something bad is going to happen…eh…
Margaret:	Yes, just stay with that. Do you feel it in your body? (Jonah: Yeah) Where?
Jonah:	Yes, in my arms and a feeling in my stomach. Just feel anxious and, like, shaky, like I'm going to fail something.
Margaret:	Come over here. [Pointing to critic chair; Jonah switches chairs] Be this voice that makes him lack confidence, makes him nervous like he's going to fail.
Jonah:	It's that I feel that people look, that other people look at me while my boss is asking me to do something, and they are thinking what a fool I am.
Margaret:	Tell him here that, 'Other people look at you… Other people look at you, evaluating you'…
Jonah [as Critic]:	Yes, looking up and down at you…(gesturing) and… they stand there all looking, while I'm there sitting and it's like, 'You're stupid!' or, 'You're in trouble.'

Stage 3b. Deepening: Deepening in the Experiencer. After developing the critical voice, the counsellor concentrates on helping the client in the Experiencing chair to attend to their current primary emotional experience in response to the criticisms. Turning attention inside (again a form of focusing) helps clients get past their initial secondary reactive emotions and move towards their deeper, more primary feelings (see Chapter 2). By helping the client refine each aspect and access underlying feelings, the counsellor allows contact and negotiation between the two sides to take place:

Margaret:	Will you change. (Jonah switches chairs.) What do you feel inside right now?
Jonah [as Experiencer]:	Well, I feel tight, anxious, and I feel tired.
Margaret:	Yeah, it's exhausting having this voice always at you.
Jonah:	I get tired of always being on guard, alert.

Margaret:	Uh-huh. You sound tired. Tell him. Tell him what it's like for you. [promoting responsibility]
Jonah:	He doesn't care. [bitter laugh]
Margaret:	Uh-huh. Leaves you feeling uncared for.
Jonah:	Yeah!
Margaret:	Tell him about it. [promoting responsibility]
Jonah:	I feel pressured, demanded on, and I feel uncared for. [pause]
Margaret:	So what are you experiencing as you say this? [Exploratory question to access feelings]
Jonah:	Stuck [sighs]. I'm tired all the time, and I never have the chance to rejuvenate.
Margaret:	So what are you saying to him? What do you want or need? [Encourage recognition of need]
Jonah:	I want... I want, basically I want to rest.
Margaret:	Tell him again.
Jonah:	Basically, keep quiet. Leave me alone. Shut up.
Margaret:	What do you need from him?
Jonah:	I need you to cut me some slack, to stop pressuring, watching, warning. I need support, not criticism.

Stage 3c. Deepening: Specifying core negative treatment of self. As the client goes back and forth between the two aspects/chairs, the counsellor continues to help the client to become more aware of specific self-criticisms and injunctions ('shoulds'). The focus here is on becoming more concrete and specific. Thus, when the critic says, 'You should work harder', the counsellor offers a process suggestion: 'Can you be more specific? What should he do specifically? Tell him.' This facilitates the client's next statement, 'Last night you shouldn't have given up at 10:30. You should have stuck with it at least another hour.' The change from the global 'should' to the more specific complaints begins to reveal much more of the idiosyncratic content and quality of the person's self-criticisms.

The counsellor also brings the client's attention to their Critic's manner and style, helping the client to become aware not only of *what* is being said, but also of *how* this is occurring. This is explicated as fully as possible by enacting the manner, such as being harsh, scolding or guilt-producing. The counsellor thus helps the dialogue unfold by listening carefully to both the content and style of each aspect as expressed by the client and makes explicit both the 'what' and the 'how' of the self-criticisms.

An important aim is to help the client articulate their core criticism. The counsellor might direct the client to repeat and exaggerate phrases or nonverbal expressions associated with self-disapproval. For example, if the client says 'you're worthless' or sneers while criticizing, the counsellor directs the client to 'do this again...', 'do this some more...', 'put some words to this...'. This helps access core criticisms and intensifies the client's emotional arousal.

Note that the Experiencing self's emotions often emerge first in the Critic chair as emotional pain is triggered by heightened self-attack. In this case, it's important for the counsellor to recognize that the pain belongs to the self-experiencer, sometimes waiting for an appropriate moment to ask the client to switch.

Stage 3d. Deepening: Continuing to access and express underlying feelings in Experiencer and Critic. The counsellor continues to use a focusing process to help the client to access and deepen primary feelings, guiding them to focus inwards and attend to emotion or by asking the client to express feelings to the Critic. The counsellor might enquire: 'What do you experience in your body?' The client's response, 'I feel defeated', is then responded to with a reflection of the client's feelings, for example, of hopelessness. This reflection is followed by a process suggestion that the client express this feeling to the other chair in order to activate more feeling and to keep the focus on the dialogue between the parts rather than on speaking to the counsellor. The counsellor tracks the feelings as they change, focuses on the emerging new experience, and encourages both the exploration and expression of the emerging experience. The counsellor promotes active expression of feelings. The counsellor thus might say, 'Tell him what you feel', suggesting the expression of the feeling to the other chair, or saying, 'What do you want to say to that side?'

After this, the therapist has Jonah go back to the Critic chair to continue the dialogue:

Margaret:	Change. (Jonah moves to Critic chair) Then what happens next? What does this part say to him? I guess this is where you dump on yourself, is it? OK, so what else… what do you say, 'You screwed up'?
Jonah:	Yeah.
Margaret:	Big time! 'You're a loser'.
Jonah:	Yeah, that's right.
Margaret:	Say it. [heightening the Critic]
Jonah:	You're a loser.
Margaret:	What else, how else do you dump?… I mean do you see that you are continually dumping on him?
Jonah:	Aah…You're hopeless. [Brushing off gesture towards other chair.]
Margaret:	What is this? [The counsellor is enquiring about the client's hand gesture]. You are kind of quite scornful of… and also dismissing of… you're quite despairing… when you throw up your hands in despair with him and giving up on him with this scorn and kind of 'Ahh! You're not even worth… bothering with any more.' [turning process into content]
Jonah:	Yes, that's right.
Margaret:	So do this then. Be scornful and kind of dismissive – do it.
Jonah:	Uh huh… you're hopeless. You are… [pauses] pathetic.

Stage 4. Emerging shift: Primary underlying feelings and needs emerge. At this point, the core negative view of self has been reached, along with the pain associated with it. Jonah's counsellor offered him the chance to move to the next stage by having him move back to the Experiencer chair to express the core pain and the need that comes with it:

Margaret:	Change chairs. [Jonah switches] Now from over here stay with the feeling. How do you feel when you get this?
Jonah:	Well, it is awful, but I… Yeah, it feels awful, it feels terrible.

Margaret:	Tell him about how awful it feels… crushing or…?
Jonah:	Yeah, it is paralyzing. I feel terrified and ashamed [choking sound]
Margaret:	It is paralyzing and just totally immobilizes you, it freezes you. So painful. (Jonah: Mhm). Mhm. So: 'I can't move and you've got me locked in a corner'? What is happening inside? Your eyes are looking really tortured…
Jonah:	I am feeling very tortured. Powerless. Humiliated, unable to do anything for myself.
Margaret:	What do you need?
Jonah:	(Sighs) I don't know. I guess I need him to treat me better. It's also like, 'Stop it, back off'?
Margaret:	What do you feel right now?
Jonah:	Angry, pissed off, like, 'Stop it, back off, leave me alone.'
Margaret:	Say it again.
Jonah:	Yeah, stop doing that.
Margaret:	And back off.
Jonah:	And back off.

This is an important shift as the client has become aware of, labelled, and expressed his anger and more assertive feelings. He has also set limits with the Critic and told his Critic to stop being so critical. In a later dialogue the client was able to further set limits with the Critic and to ask for support and encouragement. This Critic agreed to be more reassuring and supportive and less critical.

What has happened here? An issue of crucial importance in this stage of the dialogue is how one works with the painful feelings in the Experiencing chair. Clients will experience and express intense feelings of sadness, despair, insecurity, exhaustion, and inadequacy, among others. How do we respond, and how do we facilitate change in these feelings? When the client enters a painful state, saying, 'I feel weak' or 'I feel sad', the counsellor helps the client stay with the feeling rather than moving away from it. They ask the client to immerse fully in the feeling by suggesting, 'Stay with your sadness', or 'Let it come, speak from it', or 'Can you put some words to your feeling?'. Essentially, this helps the client direct as much attention as possible to the experience in order to identify with it as fully as possible, and to symbolize it as accurately as possible. Once claimed as one's own and symbolized, the painful feelings are further differentiated and developed into phrases such as 'I'm afraid life is passing me by', 'I feel all alone and soft', or 'I feel exposed and vulnerable'. This involves the client coming to new meaning through both discovery and creation. Experience is symbolized and new possibilities are created. The client's growth tendency and the counsellor's empathic attunement to it leads to forward movement.

A key counsellor intervention, following the identification and symbolizing of feelings, is the asking of exploratory questions that enquire into the client's experience, particularly their needs and wants. This facilitates elaboration and differentiation. It is useful to note that the question, 'What's it like inside?', asked in an exploratory tone, is more effective in facilitating symbolization than 'What are you feeling?' The former question promotes differentiated bottom-up description, whereas the latter can lead to conceptual, top-down labelling and so is used less often.

This process of differentiation of feeling leads to new experiences and needs associated with emergent feelings. Thus, the experience 'I'm afraid' or 'I feel vulnerable' may evolve into 'I feel delicate, and I like this feeling' when new features of the experience are attended to. Furthermore, when the feeling 'I feel unworthy' differentiates into 'I did my best, but it wasn't enough for you', it may then transform further into 'I feel angry' and finally into the assertion to the other chair: 'You expect too much of me.' Given that emotions are action tendencies, once the emerging emotion has been identified, it is crucial to identify the action tendency and need associated with it. 'I feel exhausted' generally contains within it a tendency to pull back or cease effort and a need to relax. 'I feel angry' generally contains a thrusting forward and a need to defend or break free. However, it is important to note that all human experiences are ultimately idiosyncratic. There are different types of exhaustion and anger for different people and different types for the same person at different times. Thus, each feeling needs to be explored for its current unique action tendency and need.

When a client's pain or basic insecurity has been contacted in the Experiencer, any tendency to move away from this discomfort is overcome by support from the counsellor and the collaborative therapeutic alliance to stay with this painful feeling in order to accept it and allow it to develop. The person might experience feeling shaky and unsafe, feeling existentially vulnerable – afraid of falling apart, or of collapsing, disappearing or becoming chaotic. However, this is not an out-of-control, panic state. It is an allowing, experiencing process in which the person is facing their core pain, most basic fear, or most fundamental insecurity. This is done in the safety of the presence of another, who provides the acceptance and the security that helps the person to feel contained. Having allowed the pain or insecurity and experienced it in this safety, a transformational process occurs in which the person contacts his or her own inner resources, organismic capacities, and confidence. Paradoxically, this often occurs by owning and confidently asserting 'I feel unsure' or 'Yes, I do feel terrified'. From this congruent and self-accepting base of feeling what is, be that insecurity or vulnerability or pain, the person begins to feel more able to cope. It has been the struggle against this feeling that has utilized so much of the person's internal resources and attention and that has kept the person weak and split. The acceptance of the feeling by allowing it, and discovering that one survives the feeling, frees up internal resources that can be used to enhance coping with the *world* rather than coping with the *self*. It is this type of acknowledgement and expression of the organism's primary feelings that makes it possible for the Critic to shift out of the self-blame.

Softening/Negotiation and Postdialogue Stages

Stage 5: Softening and negotiation. At a later point in the dialogue, the values and standards underlying the Critic sometimes emerge. The counsellor helps the Critic now express what has been motivating the criticisms. Sometimes it is the person's intrinsic hope and ideals. Now values and standards like, 'I've always wanted to become a doctor', may emerge. This is an intrinsic value, not an extrinsic one such as, 'My mother wants me to become a doctor', which is an introject (an internalization of something from someone else).

After the shift in the experiencing part, negotiation or integration can be facilitated between the two aspects of self by the client shuttling back and forth between the two aspects and having each express their own perspectives and needs. Sometimes it is useful for the counsellor to facilitate explicit negotiation between the parts; at other times, a new integration spontaneously emerges and only needs the counsellor to help to consolidate it. The client often will begin to experience a coming together of the two aspects, as though the differences between them have melted into a single more unified perspective. An example of a negotiated integration is given below, taken from Jonah's counselling:

Margaret:	Uh-huh ... So over here. [Jonah switches chairs.]
Jonah [as Experiencer]:	[chuckles] Well, you see, but I want to run off with stars in my eyes. [laughs] That's the whole point. [laughs] Um... I think you've missed the whole thing... um... I don't mind you watching me, and I don't mind you making... you know, comments, and, I don't mind you... bringing up things... but you can be such a wet blanket.
Margaret:	Uh-huh [laughs].
Jonah:	And I really don't want you around. Well, I want you – No, that's not altogether true. I want you to be there... for me to call on if I need you... but stop being such a wet blanket.
Margaret:	So what do you want from him? [Facilitate negotiation]
Jonah:	When you see I'm about to make... some disastrous decision, then you could step in. But for the rest of the time, let me... let me breathe (Margaret: Uh-huh) Give me room. Don't stifle me.

Through the transcripts of Jonah's sessions, we have seen the Critic soften into both fear and compassion and end in a type of negotiation between the two sides. However, if the Critic is an introject from abusive or rejecting others, it will remain hostile and not soften. Especially with very destructive Critics, there will be no standards and values to express, and the process will move to a boundary setting process where the self gets rid of the introjected voice by standing up to it and rejecting it from a position of self-worth and strength.

Stage 6: Postdialogue creation of meaning. In the postdialogue stage, when appropriate, the counsellor and the client reflect on the client's in-session experience to *create meaning.* Thus, after the dialogue, having checked how the client is feeling, the client is asked what sense they make of what happened in the dialogue. The counsellor will also say how they saw what happened (*empathic formulation*) and might use this as a time for *experiential teaching*, which is teaching by describing or explaining something the client experienced in the session. This is 'hot teaching' because it is based on lived emotional experience that has just happened rather than more cold experience of distanced, more rational explanation. More importantly, client and therapist will collaborate on developing a shared understanding or story of how the client's process works ('case formulation') and how to move forward.

When a resolution has not been reached, the counsellor may summarize by using empathic formulation responses to help create a shared story of the client's process. For example, the counsellor might say:

> *Margaret:* So I guess that's the big dilemma for you; there really are these two kind of voices in you. (Jonah: Yeah, absolutely.) One is this really harsh critical part that leaves the other part never feeling good enough. (Jonah: Mmhm), and then somehow you try to make up for that by trying to be… (Jonah: Perfect) Yeah, perfect. And then you tie yourself in knots and end up feeling so overwhelmed. Does that fit? (Jonah: Yeah, that pretty much sums it up.)

The counsellor may also offer *awareness homework* related to discoveries in the dialogue (Greenberg & Warwar, 2006; Warwar & Ellison, 2019). Homework can be given, such as suggesting that during the week the client become aware of, for example, the critical voice and its impact, or the manner the person adopts in delivering internal criticisms, or the experiencing self's feelings and needs. In addition to becoming aware, the counsellor can suggest that the client deliberately engage in any of the above processes during the week. This is done to bring them into awareness and under control by turning automatic processing into controlled processing (Greenberg & Safran, 1984, 1987).

Working with Other Kinds of Conflicts

In this chapter, we have emphasized self-critical splits, the most important, fundamental kind. However, as noted earlier, there are many variant types of conflict, all slightly different from one another (see Table 6.1). For example, in *motivational or self-damaging splits*, clients may be pushing the self to do something like work harder but find that they are procrastinating instead. This kind of conflict often starts out in a rather intellectualized or superficial manner, and generally needs the counsellor to help the client to access an underlying harsh critical voice and a rebellious experiencer.

On the other hand, *self-interruption splits* arise when one part of the self blocks or constricts emotional experience and expression, as when the client says, 'I can feel the tears coming up, but I just tighten and suck them back in. Somehow I just can't let myself cry.' Two chair work with this kind of split has in the past been referred to as *two chair enactment* (Elliott et al., 2004) because the emphasis is on making the interrupting part of the self explicit by turning the automatic process of interruption into a deliberate one. Self-interruption is essentially giving oneself the instruction 'Don't feel, don't need, don't speak', but also involves complex, physiological, muscular, emotional processes that inhibit experience and expression. Blocks range from dissociation to stifling tears to changing the subject. Resignation and deadness are often the result of squashing and suppressing emotions. 'What's the use' often captures this feeling. In working with self-interruptions, the process first involves helping clients become aware *that* they are blocking, and then *how* they are blocking. This enables them to become aware of their agency in the process of blocking their emotions. This in the long run helps them allow the emotional experience that is avoided.

In comparison to self-critical splits, markers of self-interruptive splits typically have a largely nonverbal, bodily aspect; sometimes they are purely nonverbal, such as a head-ache or tightness in the chest and may be completely automatic. The therapist's goals in self-interruptive work are both to heighten awareness of agency in the interruptive pro-cess and to help the client access and allow blocked or disavowed internal experience.

Bethany: Two Chair Work in the Early Working Phase

In Chapter 5, we saw Bethany and Robert using unfolding and focusing in session 3 to access her guarding and self-critical internal voices. Picking up the process from this point, the counsellor moves into experiential teaching, explaining how EFC works with these different voices, the guarding and critical ones. Bethany says she generally tries to block them out. Because it's only session 3, the counsellor discloses that he's now wondering if she's ready to start working on these voices using the chairs. Bethany reports feeling open to this, so the counsellor explains that making the voices explicit takes away some of their power and that the chairs can help make distance. Bethany says she's up for it.

The counsellor then uses evocative unfolding to help Bethany move into the two chair dialogue. He has her remember her experience as she came into the session today, and then asks her to change chairs and speak from the guarding part:

Bethany [as Guard/Critic]:	'You better think of something to talk about'… Then when I think of something, it says, 'That's not safe, and that's not safe, and that…'
Robert:	Be specific, what specifically isn't safe to say?
Bethany:	How you feel about myself… also your previous conversational failures… and also two more things: your mom, because we talked about that last week, so that would be boring, or your mother-in-law. Also, the way you respond to uncertainty about the future, because that's not social anxiety. No, don't talk about any of those things!
Robert:	Can you change chairs?
Bethany:	[switches chairs; as Experiencer:] But I need to have something to talk about.
Robert [gesturing to other chair]:	Change. [Bethany switches chairs.] Show me how you put pressure on her.

Bethany [as Guard/Critic]:	You have to talk about something… but don't talk about the wrong thing. [turning to counsellor, as Experiencer:] It's a lose-lose situation.
Robert:	Tell her, show me what you were telling yourself.
Bethany:	Keep thinking, find something to talk about.
Robert:	Change. [Bethany switches chairs.] What happens inside when you get this, 'Keep thinking, find something'?
Bethany [as Experiencer]:	I feel stressed. Time is running out… Then I give up: Let's get a cup of coffee!
Robert:	Is that what happens? (Bethany: Yeah) So it left you empty handed and hurting.
Bethany:	Yeah.

In this session, the unfolding, focusing and two chair tasks are used to begin the main work of counselling. Resolution is not expected at this point; instead, the client is becoming more aware of how her social anxiety process works, and most importantly beginning a process of emotional deepening.

As counselling continues, Bethany comes back to two chair work on her self-critical process in session 5. In the process she narrates more deeply about her traumatic experiences with her mother when she was a teenager, finally confessing that the core of her social anxiety is her experience of feeling that she is fundamentally malicious, selfish and harmful to others. They come back to two chair work in sessions 7 and 8, this time addressing her self-interruption process of tuning out painful experiences, as well as how she makes herself anxious (this is an anxiety split), and the underlying self-critical process. Along the way, they continue building up an experience-based story of how Bethany's various difficult experiences fit together to make her anxious and unhappy in her life. This process thus occupies much of the client's counselling and provides the groundwork needed for other kinds of work (see Chapters 7 and 8) that will enable her to transform her primary maladaptive fear, guilt, and shame about damaging others, helping her replace them with more adaptive self-caring and compassion.

Further Exploration

Reading

Elliott, R., Watson, J. C., Goldman, R. N., & Greenberg, L. S. (2004). *Learning emotion-focused therapy: The process-experiential approach to change.* Washington, DC: American Psychological Association. [See Chapter 11]

Greenberg, L. S., & Watson, J.C. (2005). *Emotion-focused therapy of depression.* Washington, DC: American Psychological Association. [See Chapter 10]

Shahar, B., Carlin, E. R., Engle, D. E., Hegde, J., Szepsenwol, O., & Arkowitz, H. (2012). A pilot investigation of emotion-focused two-chair dialogue intervention for self-criticism. *Clinical Psychology & Psychotherapy*, 19(6), 496–507. Online first, 28 June 2011. doi: 10.1002/cpp.762

Watson, J., Goldman, R., & Greenberg, L. S. (2007). *case studies in emotion-focused therapy for depression*. Washington, DC: American Psychological Association. [Try enacting transcripts throughout]

Watching

Greenberg, L. S. (2004). *Emotion-Focused Therapy of Depression*. American Psychological Association videos [See session 1 for demonstration of self-critical dialogue]

Greenberg, L. S. (2008). *Emotion-Focused Therapy over Time*. American Psychological Association videos. [See session 2 for demonstration of two chair work for self-interruption split]

Greenberg, L. S. (2020). *Emotion-Focused Therapy: Working with Core Emotion*. Counselling Channel video. [Two chair self-interruption work, plus other processes]

Reflecting

1. Identify a conflict you have experienced between two parts of you, where one part of you caused you stress or made you feel bad. After writing a brief description of this experience, look at Table 6.1 and see if you can identify what kind of conflict split it was. (Hint: It could be more than one at the same time.)
2. Silently to yourself, put words to your critical voice and then imagine yourself in front of you and say them to yourself. See how this makes you feel and tell the critic how you feel. Identify the most painful feeling you have in reaction to your critic and then ask yourself what you need from the critic instead of the criticism.
3. If you were using two chair work with a client, what might you do to make the work more collaborative and less something you impose on the client?

7

Late Working Phase: Empty Chair Work for Unresolved Relational Issues

---

Chapter Outline

Overview of Empty Chair Work

Task Initiation and Entry Stages of Empty Chair Work

Heightening and Expressing Stages of Empty Chair Work

Completing and Processing Stages of Empty Chair Work

Variations in Empty Chair Work

Further Exploration

Overview of Empty Chair Work

In this chapter we move deeper into the working phase of EFC by describing the other major form of chair work in EFC: Empty Chair work for unresolved relational issues ('unfinished business'), giving steps and showing you how Jonah used this task in his counselling. In the next chapter we briefly present two related tasks, *Empathic Affirmation* and *Compassionate Self-soothing*, another form of chair work; at that point we will also pick up with the late working phase of Bethany's counselling. These tasks emerge increasingly as the working phase of EFC progresses and the client moves towards their core pain.

Borrowing from psychodrama (Moreno & Moreno, 1959), empty chair work was developed in Gestalt therapy (Perls et al., 1951) to assist clients in processing their unresolved emotions and in finding new ways to come to terms with past hurts and unresolved grief, instead of dwelling on them in unproductive ways. We have studied and refined this process as a means to help clients come to terms with emotional injuries that happened primarily in the past.

When hurtful others are no longer available to be spoken to, or have distanced themselves from the client or made it clear that they are unwilling to hear what their past behaviour has done to the client, the client still can be helped by engaging in a dialogue with the imagined other, as if the other person were in the counselling room, sitting in an empty chair. Alternatively, when a client feels they have in some way let down an important other who has died or can no longer be contacted, it can be very useful to help them to say to the imagined other in the session what they were unable to say directly. This enables the client to get in touch with their internal view of the other person. Client and counsellor together create a virtual reality in which memories are activated and can be reconsolidated with new input, changing the person's experience of the past. Previously disowned feelings and unmet needs are experienced and voiced, allowing the emotions to be symbolized and the needs and action tendencies associated with them to be completed. Moreover, the counsellor helps the client through an emotional deepening process that ultimately enables the client to access new feelings that change the old feelings and helps them create a new story about self and the other. This in turn enables clients to step back from the relationship (whether remembered or currently ongoing) and recognize the legitimacy of their needs. This also helps free the client from old stuck bad feelings and the hope that the other will apologize or that things will be put right. When it is successful, empty chair work leads to shifts in views of both self and the other. This can lead to understanding, forgiveness or holding the other accountable for wrongs done; in particular, it helps the person let go of trying to get the other to meet that need, and to begin to explore which of their other meaningful relationships or projects might meet their needs. The steps of the dialogue are outlined in Table 7.1 and described in detail below.

TABLE 7.1   *Empty chair work for unresolved relational issues: Task resolution model*

Task Resolution Stage	Counsellor Responses

1. *Task Initiation*:
 	
   1a. *Marker*: Blames, complains, or expresses hurt or longing in relation to a significant other.
   1b. *Align* to offered task
	• Listen for, reflect towards possible unfinished business markers (including during other tasks, e.g., two chair dialogue).
	• Establish collaboration and structure experiment.
	• Obtain client agreement by offering experiential teaching, experiential formulation related to task.

2. *Entering*:
 	
   2a. *Making psychological contact* with other
   2b. *Speaking directly* in first person to imagined other and expressing unresolved feelings
	• Evoke the sensed presence of the significant other.
	• Access client's initial feelings in response to the significant other.
	• Encourage speaking directly to significant other.
	• Facilitate the taking of responsibility (first-person language).
	• *As needed: Listen for and help client to deal with difficulties engaging in task.*

Task Resolution Stage	Counsellor Responses

3. **Heightening**:
 	
  3a. *Evoking* increasingly strong feelings towards other via enacting other/episodic memories
 	
  3b. *Differentiating* complaint into underlying primary feelings
 	
  3c. *Resolving self-interruptions*
	• *As needed: Facilitate enactment of the significant other and intensify the stimulus value of the significant other.*
	• Evoke a specifically recalled event or episodic memory.
	• Differentiate feelings towards significant other.
	• *As needed: Listen for, help client to work with emergent self-interruptive processes.*
	• *When approaching end of session without resolution, help client to close contact and formulate what has been learned so far.*

4. **Expressing**:
 	
  4a. *Reaching moderately* high levels of emotional expression
 	
  4b. Experiencing *unmet needs* as valid and expressing them assertively
	• Promote full expression to significant other of differentiated primary/adaptive emotion by graded experiments of expression.
	• Help to maintain a balance between expression and contact with inner experience.
	• Facilitate expression to significant other of unfulfilled needs and expectations.
	• Provide empathic affirmation for emerging unmet needs.

5. **Completing: Letting go of unresolved feelings and needs**:
 	
  5a. *Other resolution work*: Coming to understand and see other in a new way; understanding, forgiving, or holding other accountable
 	
  5b. *Self-resolution work*: Affirming self; exploring appropriate ways to meet unmet needs.
	• Identify with/enact other and support emerging new representation of other.
	• Support emerging new understanding of other and of relationship with other.
	• Offer support for forgiveness, understanding or holding other accountable.
	• Support/affirm client to validate self.
	• Support client in exploring appropriate ways to meet unmet need.

6. **Post-chair work processing**:
 	
  6a. *Transitioning* out of chair work
 	
  6b. *Appreciating*/dwelling on emerging self-affirmation/ empowerment
 	
  6c. Developing *meaning perspective*/shared formulation/narrative
	• Close contact with the other appropriately.
	• Help client to appreciate emerging self-affirmation.
	• Help client to create meaning perspective/shared formulation/narrative.

Empty chair work versus two chair attribution split work. Before we go any further, here is a tricky bit: there are actually two different ways of working with other people in the empty chair. The first and most common of these is *unfinished business work* (UFB for short), which is our main focus here. In unfinished business work, the other in the empty chair is a specific other giving the negative message the client experienced in the relationship. In UFB, it's a case of the client having particular unresolved feelings and specific emotion memories with the other, especially feelings of shame or unmet longings that are central in the distress, for example, 'I'm carrying this feeling towards you'.

The other way of working with other people is *attribution split* work, mentioned in the previous chapter. This involves the client playing an introjection (internalized image) of a specific other (e.g., a parent) or generalized other or kind of other (e.g., bullies, oppressors). In attribution split work, this internalized voice of the other is understood to be an aspect of the client and is enacted in the other chair. In attribution splits, it is the parent's internalized voice in the client's head that is being worked with. The client may have internalized a negative message (e.g., 'You'll never amount to anything') and now says this to self. In other words, attribution splits involve being colonized by the other (a kind of internalised oppression), while in UFB it is the specific painful emotional memories and the unresolved sadness, anger, etc. that are troubling, not the parent's voice in their heads. The person is pained by actual experiences that led to emotional injuries to attachment and identity. Sometimes when the parent is in the empty chair, it is a bit unclear which process is engaged! Fortunately, you don't need to know definitely which it is to start, because this will clarify as you work. When there is no specific *episodic* memory of the other engaging in the action, but rather the client has a *generic* memory that formed across situations and is now part of their inner critic, then we are working with an introjected other. On the other hand, unfinished business is the client feeling sad and angry at specific past hurts. In our experience, splits and unfinished business are often intertwined, but one aspect generally is more salient than the other.

Task Initiation and Entry Stages of Empty Chair Work

Stage 1. Task initiation. Empty chair work can be used for just about any type of unresolved relational issue in the client's life, past or present. However, it is most effective with the signature marker of *unfinished business*, defined as stuck, unresolved bad feelings from past interactions with an important person in our life (a significant other). A clear give-away of this marker is recurrent experiences of pain, anger, sadness, and vulnerability that we feel every time we are reminded of what happened in the past or think about the person who hurt us or left us. The marker involves a statement of a lingering, unresolved feeling towards an important other, stated in a highly involved manner, for example:

> Client: My father, he just was never there for me. I have never forgiven him; deep down inside I think I'm somehow grieving for what I probably didn't have and know I never will have.

We will discuss two variant markers later, trauma-related unfinished business and current conflictual relationships, which require somewhat different handling.

Stage 2. Entering. When clients show that they are ready to work on their unresolved past wounds, it's useful to provide empathic affirmation for these feelings and then to move towards setting up a dialogue. At the beginning, it's important to ensure that the client is making contact with the imagined other: you can ask the client to imagine the other in the empty chair. Evoking the sensed presence of the other, making sure the person is currently experiencing the imagined presence of the person, in a direct and immediate way, is important for evoking both relevant episodic memories and associated more general emotion schemes connected with the other. You might introduce a dialogue with process suggestions:

- I wonder if we could bring her in here and tell her this. Maybe not what you tell her in real life but what you wish you could say, your truth.
- I hear that you have a lot of lingering feelings towards him. Let's try something… can you put him in the chair. (pause) Just picture him sitting over there. What do you feel when you see him?

Once client and counsellor have got into the chair work and are working together on the task, such long process suggestions will get in the client's way, so it's a good idea to switch to brief commands, like 'Tell her', as a kind of shorthand to encourage the client to express feelings to the other. (Some counsellors may be put off by this, but really it's like two people working together to move a large wardrobe.)

Jonah. As the sessions progressed, Jonah revealed that he felt worthless and ashamed as a result of his mother's denigration of him when he was a child. As a consequence of growing up with a mother who ridiculed his feelings and was abusive and threatening, he was afraid of rejection. He felt misunderstood by his mother and had learned that his feelings were dangerous. Thus, an important focus of therapy became for him to resolve his abuse-related unfinished business with his mother. However, in order to do this, he first needed help with allowing and tolerating his feelings, which he was used to pushing away. As the counsellor empathically explored his feelings about his relationship with his mother over the sessions, Jonah began to express how angry he was at her, and also how hopeless he was that she would ever change. In an attempt to help Jonah to activate some of his feelings towards his mother, his counsellor Margaret introduced empty chair work in session 8. As Jonah began to express his anger to the counsellor, he became afraid and ashamed that he could not do anything about how he had been treated.

Margaret:	Mm-hm, let-, let's try something. This is sometimes very helpful. (Jonah: OK) You've been telling me what you wish you could say to her. What I'd like you to do is to just imagine for a moment that your mom is sitting there, can you see her there? … Something is happening? [Process suggestions to structure the task]
Jonah:	(sigh) … (sigh)
Margaret:	Lots of big sighs [Process reflection]

Jonah:	I've just been calming down (chuckle)
Margaret:	So what was it you're... what are you trying to calm? Just imagining her there brings up a lot of feelings doesn't it? [exploratory question followed by empathic conjecture]
Jonah:	(sigh) (pause)
Margaret:	What are you trying to do? [exploratory question]
Jonah:	Oh, I guess the usual; take control of the situation internally, um ... trying to look at the other side of the situation of it, um...
Margaret:	OK so let's just – you don't have to go too fast, I'm just curious, what happens when I say 'Imagine her sitting there'? Cause I could see, lots of stuff is happening... How would she be if she was sitting there? What does she look like?
Jonah:	If she was sitting there now? (Sniff) um (sigh) defiant. (pause)
Margaret:	So what do you feel inside when you see her defiantly over there.
Jonah (in a flat tone):	I feel scared.

Note the use of exploratory questions and process reflections to help Jonah to get started on the task.

Heightening and Expressing Stages of Empty Chair Work

Stage 3. Heightening. Having helped the client enter into the process of making psychological contact and speaking directly to the other, the next step is to help them begin to evoke and express their feelings more strongly towards the other. There are several issues to be aware of during this stage of the work, both strategies for helping clients heighten their emotions and the difficulties that can emerge.

Balance empathy with process guiding. As a basic style, follow a reflection with a process suggestion. For example, the counsellor might respond to the client in the self chair with 'Feeling really hesitant' (= reflection), then follow this with 'Tell her again, "I'm hesitant to say this"' (= process suggestion).

Enacting the negative other. Although it sounds counter-intuitive, it can be very useful to have the client be the other person, performing the hurtful behaviour that is so difficult for the client. This helps to evoke an emotional reaction in the client, particularly if they are having trouble accessing their feelings. We are asking the client to do something that the other did that drove the client crazy or hurt them. Enacting the other in their negative mode evokes the client's emotional reaction to them. You can ask the client what the other said or did specifically, and then ask the client to do this. It's useful to get the details of the insults, acts of neglect or hurtful behaviours towards the client. The point of enacting the significant other is not to have a debate between self and other in the chairs, but instead to arouse emotions. It is important to evoke the client's feelings in the self chair and to tease apart the different causes of the injury. The other can be enacted a number of times to evoke more feeling.

When a client is enacting the other in the empty chair in order to get a sense of the impact of the other on the self, you can ask, 'What was the message she gave you? What did her face or voice say?' It's useful not to get too caught up in the specific content of the client's narrative, which can easily take you and the client away from the emotions. Instead, it's a good idea to stay attuned to the emotional tone that is evident in what the client says, like trying to listen to the music of the feeling in it. You can also check in with the client to determine whether they are feeling what they are saying: 'As you say this, what do you feel?'

Once the client has enacted the negative actions and attitudes of the other, the client's emotional reaction, in the self chair, becomes the focus. The client is invited to move back to the self chair and is asked, 'How do you react to that? What happens inside when you hear that from her?' With your careful and attuned tracking and reflections, relevant feelings towards the other will emerge. It is important to help clients both make contact with their feelings and use these to contact the other.

Addressing client hesitation. Clients need help both to be aware of and to express their feelings. If the client is too reluctant to face the other, it's important for you not to panic. This is normal and is completely understandable. Don't try to force them to speak directly to the other in the empty chair. Instead, be curious about their reaction and help them explore their reasons for not wanting to face the other. Feel free to be creative with the process. For example, you can turn the chair away or put it far away at first (progressive approximation to contact with the other); or you can help them identify and explore the blocks to contact. (We'll come back to this shortly when we discuss self-interruptions during empty chair work; see pp. 103–104 and Chapter 6.) But the main thing is for you to just stay with the client and be interested in what is so difficult for them about facing the other.

Dealing with undifferentiated and secondary reactive emotion responses. When clients talk about unresolved past emotional injuries, they typically first express a mix of hurt and resentment. The outrage or protest against the unfairness of what happened comes out as complaint. These are secondary reactive emotions obscuring the underlying anger and sadness. Sometimes there is a sense of defeat, resignation, and hopelessness. 'What is the use of getting worked up about it? Nothing will change.' Complaint must always be separated out into its more basic components of anger and sadness, each of which needs to be experienced, put into words, and expressed on its own. The typical secondary emotions expressed in empty chair work are hopelessness, resignation, depression, and anxiety, typically expressed in an outer-directed manner with a blaming tone, for example: 'You were a terrible parent! You never should have been allowed to have children.' Of course, it's important for the counsellor to give empathy to and help clients to work through the secondary anger, complaint or hopelessness. However, the aim is to encourage the client to directly express primary maladaptive emotions of anger and sadness, such as, 'I resent you', or 'I missed having you around', rather than, 'You were a bastard' or 'Why did you neglect me?' The fused anger and sadness of complaint often comes out in question form: 'Why couldn't you be more…?', or 'Why did you do that? I just want to know why?' It is important to help clients to move beyond these secondary reactions, beyond complaint, and past accusatory why-questions, to expressing their primary maladaptive, stuck sadness, anger, fear, and shame towards the imagined other. In cases of abuse, combinations of unresolved maladaptive fear, shame, and disgust also need to be accessed, validated, and reprocessed, to the point where the client is able to access primary adaptive anger and sadness (Greenberg, 2015).

In working with anger, it is also important, as we have pointed out in Chapter 2, to distinguish between secondary reactive and primary adaptive anger. Primary adaptive anger, or anger in response to current violation, is essential and must be validated and its expression encouraged. In unfinished business, this anger may have been blocked, pushed away or even denied at the time because it was unsafe to express it in the original relationship. When they are stuck in secondary reactive emotions (emotions about emotions), people lose access to their more direct primary responses. Even when these are stuck, maladaptive emotion responses, they are still the person's more basic experience and therefore one step closer to primary adaptive emotions, the healthy resources that can promote adaptive behaviour. Thus, the expression of anger and standing up to the other, by saying, for example, 'I am angry at you for hurting me like that. You were sick, and I did not deserve to be treated like that!' is empowering and healing. As noted in Chapter 2, to distinguish primary anger from secondary reactive anger, counsellors use the following criteria: adaptive anger (a) is in response to violation, (b) involves assertion, and (c) is empowering. In contrast, secondary reactive anger has a more blustery, destructive quality to it, serves to push the other away, or obscures the expression of more vulnerable emotion. Its expression does not bring relief or promote the working through of experience.

The counsellor at all times brings the process back to feelings with 'I feel' type statements, such as 'What are you feeling now?' or 'What feelings come up in you when she says that?' It's important to bring the client back to the present: 'What do you feel as you say this. Tell her.' Narrative statements focused on the past, such as 'I was' or 'I felt', are changed to present-oriented statements: 'I am' or 'I feel'. In addition, clients have to be encouraged to tolerate their painful emotions. It is important to help clients to accept and stay with their emotions rather than rushing too quickly to try to change them.

In Jonah's empty chair work, the counsellor helped him move into stage 3 as follows:

Margaret:	So could you come sit here for a minute? I want you to, do what she does, be her, take on that defiant kind of look at Jonah there. [process suggestion]
Jonah:	(Moves to other chair and looks) (sighs) (pause)
Margaret:	So you're looking down your nose at him? [process reflection]
Jonah:	Why don't you grow up?
Margaret:	OK, so you just, that's what she says: 'Why don't you grow up'.
Jonah:	(to counsellor:) That's frankly exactly I think what she would say.

Margaret:	OK, come back in this chair. 'Just grow up, Jonah! Whatever your problems are, just grow up'. (pause) What happens, when you hear that? [process suggestion, followed by exploratory question]
Jonah:	(sigh) I suppose for the most part em, I figure she's right.
Margaret:	What do you actually feel now, in your body, feel?
Jonah:	Well, I feel like collapsing, sort of helpless, hurt.
Margaret:	Can you tell her? [process suggestion]
Jonah:	I guess, what I would really like, is for her to realize that, (pause) I do hurt still, a lot, and she has something to do with it, at least acknowledge 'it's (pause) me', just once.
Margaret:	OK, do you want to say to her, 'You know, I still really hurt'?
Jonah:	Yeah, but she can't hear that because she can't admit that she has any responsibility.
Margaret:	Yeah, but can you just say it? Imagine her there, and just say, 'Mom, I really hurt'. [process suggestions]
Jonah:	(sigh) I really hurt.
Margaret:	Mm-hm. (pause) Can you tell her, what hurts? What hurt you?
Jonah:	I feel that I always disappointed you, never measured up. I didn't know what the rules of the game were, and was expected to excel at them, and then you made me feel that I never could.
Margaret:	So I, I feel hurt that you always (pause) made me feel 'less than', or inadequate (pause) [evocative reflection in first person]
Jonah:	I don't believe you really care.
Margaret:	Say that again: 'I don't believe you, you really-' [Process suggestion to repeat key phrase to heighten it]
Jonah:	I don't believe you really cared about me. (sighs, begins to cry)
Margaret:	That hurts? [empathic conjecture]
(handing client the tissue box)	
Jonah:	(sigh) She told me one time when I was a kid, (sniff) 'I didn't really want to have you'.
Margaret:	Wow. Oh, that one really hurts, doesn't it? [empathic affirmation]
Jonah:	Yeah.

Self-interruption. A common occurrence in Stage 3 is self-interruption of painful or frightening emotions. Because the unresolved emotions are so painful, they are dreaded and people develop many different ways to not feel them. The process of resolution, however, requires accessing the feelings in order to change them. People protect themselves from feeling the disowned experience for fear they will fall apart if they feel them; this means that people often become emotionally blocked on the path to resolution. The counsellor needs to work to help overcome the interruption (see two chair work for self-interruption splits, in Chapter 6).

Stage 4. Expressing. Once emotions have been differentiated and interruptions overcome, the emotional arousal that is a necessary precondition for resolution of the injury emerges. Emotional arousal has been found to be an important precursor of the next step towards resolution, letting go, and change in view of self and other. Without arousal, this step is far less probable (Greenberg & Malcolm, 2002). In working with emotions at this stage, counsellors need to know that once primary emotions are fully and freely expressed, they move quickly. There is now a substantial body of useful understandings about how to help clients at this critical stage of the work, the most important of which is following the spiral of anger and sadness.

Follow the anger-sadness spiral. The client is encouraged to express previously unexpressed feelings to the imagined other in the empty chair. Often this stage involves working with the two primary emotions of anger and sadness. Anger and sadness tend to follow each other in sequence and are circularly related in a tightening spiral. In sadness, attention is often directed inwards, while in anger, expression is often directed outwards. It is important to remember that anger is the 'separating' or 'boundary setting' emotion, and its effect is to empower and legitimize feelings. Sadness, on the other hand, is the 'connecting' emotion. Its effect is to receive comfort or support.

To get through the *anger* it first must be accepted. As we like to say, you can't leave a place till you arrive at it. Recognize that resignation is often an interruption of anger. Shame and fear may also arise. Anger is a major antidote for both of these emotions. Anger is often best symbolized with 'tell him what you resent' – the word 'resent' carries a flavour of the past in a way that anger does not. When working with unexpressed anger, it's useful to start with outward-focused destructive anger (for example, 'You're a jerk'), but then shift to first-person, more inwardly-based, assertive anger (for example, 'I'm angry at you for violating me', 'I resent you for that'). Asking 'What do you need?' can be used to heighten the feeling. Moving to the need also helps the client to move from destructive anger to empowered anger ('I need you to let me be my own person'). Expression to the other is often best promoted through graded experiments (building up to the expression of intense feelings using gradual steps). You can also help the client to pump up the expression by having them say it again, louder; sometimes you can help the client override a block to expression by intensification ('Tell her, "I'm furious"'; 'Tell her again').

With *sadness*, it is best to say 'Tell him what you missed/how you were hurt'. You are looking for primary emotions in order to mobilize the need. Validate the hurt, even when the anger is there. Finally, when primary sadness is fully expressed, primary adaptive anger can emerge rapidly and help create boundaries. Conversely, the full expression of adaptive anger allows clients to acknowledge the pain of losses and betrayal and fully grieve for what they missed.

Help clients reach and maintain useful levels of emotional intensity. Remember that the counsellor's tone of voice used in empathic attunement is important. However, it is not always gentle. It must match the client's emotion. If anger is the emotion being highlighted, then the attuned voice should have an intensity to it, especially when giving directions for the expression of anger, such as 'Tell her, I resent...' with some volume and emphasis.

If the intensity of affect/experiencing wanes in the self chair, it's a good idea for the client to take the part of the other briefly in order to re-stimulate the emotion. Help them to spend time enacting the negative other, highlighting what's negative so it becomes clearer what the insult/injury/offence is. Get to the nature or the quality of the betrayal or violation. It may not be what was said that hurt so much, but *how* it was said. If it's 'disdain' or 'no concern', ask for an example. 'What was the most painful or hurtful thing they did, the thing that most gets to you even now?' Get at the meta-message delivered by the other, that is, the message about the message. Use the other as a *stimulator* of emotion, not as a debater. It may also be sufficient merely to ask the client in the self chair what the other looks like right now, including facial expression and body posture, in order to re-evoke the emotion. Ask: 'What does his face look like now? What would he say to that?' Pay attention to what appears most alive to the client at the present moment and follow and heighten that.

Stay with present experience. Interventions should elicit a present-tense stance. Don't ask questions about the past; instead, bring the client into the present to evoke feeling now. Link the content/story with the feeling in the moment, focusing on the latter, for example, 'How are you feeling now as you tell this story?', 'What's happening in your body?' Then direct the client to express this to the other. It is true that all emotions are embedded in an important story; all important stories are based on significant emotions (Angus & Greenberg, 2011). It is also true that people in general are more used to staying in a narrative mode, where the focus is on story over emotion. In EFC, however, we want to privilege the emotion over the story (but not at the expense of the story). By doing this, we are helping the client to enact the story, and in so doing, to open the possibility of creating a new story through the emotional deepening process we laid out in Chapter 3.

Focus on process more than content. Generally, 'why' questions don't deepen experience. 'How' and 'what' questions are better. An advantage of using chair dialogue is that it adds the expressive dimensions; it brings out 'the how', such as timid or hostile. Track the emotional process and the manner of expression more than the content. Notice how the client is expressing, then turn the process into content. In other words, ask 'As you're doing this, are you aware of how are you saying it?' or 'What are you expressing by your manner right now?' Pay attention to body language. How the person delivers the message is often the key message. For example, if the manner of the client is contemptuous, then direct the client to tell the other, 'I feel contempt for you'. Notice present non-verbal expressions and feed them into the dialogue, for example, if the client's hand has gone up as a shield, this may be a bodily sign that perhaps there's a need for protection from the other.

Balancing expression with inner experience. It is important to note, however, that expressing feelings, especially very dramatically, can sometimes interfere with the experience of the feeling. Therefore, after the client expresses, focus them inwards, for example,

'How does that feel, to weep?' Alternatively, after the client expresses anger, ask 'What do you feel?' (Anger and sadness can be reversed in this sequence.)

Validate feelings and needs and help clients express these directly. Evoking emotion involves not only expressing emotion but also expressing and validating the basic unmet interpersonal needs for attachment, validation or separation. These are needs that were never expressed in the original relationship because the person felt they were not entitled to do so or that their needs would not be met.

Note that intense emotional expression is more about interpersonal validation than catharsis. You don't get rid of the anger or sadness simply by expressing. You legitimize it and its intensity. Validate the legitimacy of the feeling of being wronged with interventions such as 'Tell her, I was wronged... You violated my boundaries.' Validate anger and intensify emotions by saying 'It's OK to feel anger'. At the crescendo of the anger, ask 'What did you need?' or 'Is there something you want from the other to finish this?' It is important to get a sense of whether the client's statements, such as 'I need' or 'I deserve', are grounded enough in heartfelt loss or empowered anger, or feeling of legitimacy. If not, promote empowered anger or heartfelt grief.

In order for therapy to be productive, needs must be expressed as belonging to and coming from the self, and with a sense of entitlement, rather than as protest about deprivations or as accusations of the other. Thus, they are an assertion of entitlement to the need rather than expressions of desperate neediness. This step is crucial in helping people to establish their sense of personal agency (that is, the self as an agent in their life), separate from the other, and as existing in their own right.

At this stage the counsellor encourages the expression of both emotions and needs. In addition, the counsellor helps clients to symbolize and assert boundaries, to say 'no' to intrusion, for example, or to reassert their rights. Counsellors are aware that, in early experience, people often have found it necessary to disavow their basic needs and that as a result they do not automatically attend to or express those needs. Counsellors therefore listen for needs to arise and, when they do, quickly validate them and encourage clients to express them. A thorough exploration of feelings is typically followed by a statement of related needs, as the following example shows:

Margaret:	Yeah, just this real sense of not being wanted and not being cared about and (pause) [empathic affirmation]
Jonah:	Just being a god damned pawn! (sniff). I guess that's part of, keeping it under control, cause if I ever, as I said I've only been real mad three times in my life. But not at my mother: at my wife and at work.
Margaret:	Yeah.
Jonah:	(sigh) Yeah, (sniff) I guess by bottling it all up so it kills any zest or power in life, I (pause) probably could. (sigh)
Margaret:	Mm-hm. What are you feeling, right now?
Jonah:	(sniff - sigh). Well, all kinds of things. Um, (sigh) angry, cheated, (sigh) ashamed. (pause) And the terror, and I guess, too is that, as a kid I used to feel terror.
Margaret:	What you felt was terrified, of what?

After expressing how afraid he was, he accesses his need for safety and then his anger at not having been protected. Five minutes later:

Margaret: So what did you need?

Jonah: I needed a mother who didn't beat me, terrorize me. I needed some way to feel safe.

Margaret: And what do you feel as you say this?

Jonah: I feel angry, furious. I deserved to have protection, love, a childhood free from fear.

In the above segment, the unresolved feelings of anger and sadness are expressed and the core maladaptive fear is evoked and begins to be processed. As he engaged in the task, Jonah experienced how angry he was at his mother, perhaps for the first time.

Completing and Processing Stages of Empty Chair Work

Stage 5. Completing: Letting go of unresolved feelings and needs. Strong expression of primary adaptive emotions typically leads to a new view of the self and other, although it may take several sessions to get there. Clients enter this phase when they access and directly express their key unmet needs from the other. The work then moves to helping the client feel entitled to their unmet needs, and to supporting changes in the way the client views self and other. The shift in view of the other is facilitated by emotional arousal in the self and mobilization and a sense of entitlement to previously unmet needs. Access to the need, and feeling entitled to the need, changes the person's sense of self from unworthy to worthy. Expressing the need assertively to the empty chair creates a sense of agency which transforms the previous more passive victimized experience into a more active one. Often at the heart of the injury is the fact that the trusted other either insensitively failed to recognize the hurt person's needs, or hurtfully withheld what they needed in the relationship.

Enacting the other's response to the unmet need. At this point, it is frequently useful to propose that the client enact the other. This leads to the client elaborating the world-view of the other, which aids empathy towards the injurer, while the counsellor helps the client to better understand or to hold the other accountable. A key to forgiving is developing some form of empathy towards the other. This involves seeing the world from the other's point of view and having some compassion or understanding of this view. A shift in view of the other or a new experience of the other is a very important part of the change process. In promoting a change in view of the other, work needs to be done on elaborating and understanding the world-view of the other. This work is somewhat more cognitive as it involves perspective taking and elaborating what it was like inside for the other. Taking the view of the other involves the development of empathy for the other and letting go of the expectation that the other will change.

Letting go of the unmet need. Often there is a change in view of the other that allows the need to be responded to in this virtual reality, in the therapy situation. If, however,

the imagined other is non-responsive, clients are likely to need help in grieving and letting go of wanting what they cannot get. In situations where the need cannot or will
not be met by the other, it is still important for clients to come to recognize their right
to have had their needs met by the other in the past. At this point in the dialogue, the
counsellor supports and promotes the letting go of the unfulfilled hopes and expectations. When letting go does not naturally flow from the expression of primary emotions,
counsellors can help clients explore and evaluate whether the unfulfilled expectations
can and will be met by the other, and if not, counsellors can help clients explore the
effects of hanging on to the expectations. In this situation, counsellors can consider asking clients to express to the significant other, 'I won't let you go' or 'I won't let go of the
hope you'll change'. Letting go often produces another round of grief work in which
the client works through mourning the loss of the possibility of getting the need met
from the attachment figure. This is often the most poignant and painful experience of
the process. Once the client can truly grieve, for example, for the parent they never had
or felt they let down, then they are able to let go and move on.

    Forms of resolution. Through arousal and direct expression of emotions, along with
coming to experience their needs as legitimate, clients begin to let go of narrow,
stuck views of self and others. Resolution occurs when clients are able to feel they
are worthwhile, and are able to let go of the previously unfinished bad feelings. This
letting go is accomplished in one of three major ways: (a) through holding the other
accountable for the injury experienced while also affirming the self; (b) through letting
go of the unmet need and moving on, or (c) through increased understanding of the
other, and possibly forgiving the other for past wrongs. In non-abuse cases, the client is
able to better understand the other and view the other with empathy, compassion, and,
sometimes, forgiveness. In abusive or trauma-related situations, letting go most often
involves holding the other accountable and moving on, but empathy and forgiveness
may also occur.

    Grieving the loss. The fullest form of grieving involves integrating the good aspects
of the relationship so as to be able to carry the love for the other with you after the loss.
But often anger and rage prevents this fuller grieving. This is especially true in the death
of a person who has injured you. If the internal representation of a parent who has died
remains a persecutory one of a hating or abandoning other, the parent and the loss of
what was needed can never be properly mourned. One cannot take in good that was
never there, and therefore there is no basis for forming an inner image of a good other to
live on inside. Although each bereavement and mourning process is unique to each person, it appears that mourning the loss caused by the injury is crucial. The biggest block
to the process of mourning is unresolved anger. Once the client has the experience of
the counsellor bearing witness to their anger and their suffering from the injury, their
emotional pain can decrease enough to make way for memories of the more benign or
loving aspects of the other. Even though the other has injured, abandoned, neglected
or even persecuted the self, there are generally good memories in which the other was
caring, loving, supportive or validating, and was doing the best they could. When the
client is able to retrieve these memories and become aware of the positive as well as
negative, this broadens the person's view of the other and the context. This allows the

client to move on and create a new memory and a new narrative, and allows them to see the other as more human.

Changes in the image of the other. Softening in the image of the other towards the self is an important change process in empty chair work. Research has found that this is more likely when the client is able first to express emotions at least at a moderately high level of arousal and express unmet needs in the session (Missirlian, Toukmanian, Warwar, & Greenberg, 2005). The other then often expresses guilt, shame, sorrow, regret, and compassion for the pain caused to the self. After imagining compassion in the other, the client experiences relief, soothing, grieving, letting go, and possibly forgiveness. On the other hand, in some cases the other does not soften, and the client says something like 'I'd want her to feel sorry, but she never would! She'd never get it!' Here, the counsellor could say, 'How sad it must have been for you that she is so unable to respond, that you got so little'. This generally helps clients to access more feelings to reprocess, and also begins to provide soothing through counsellor empathy and compassion.

When it does occur, the shift in the other can happen on one of two major dimensions: affiliation and power. First, there can be a shift from a neglectful other towards a more affiliative, loving other; second, the image of the other can shift from powerful to being weak and pathetic. The latter is often the case when the other has been abusive, where the client says 'Now that I'm an adult, I can see what kind of a sick person you really were'. Here, sensing that the other is less powerful is empowering to the client. So the shifts are either on an affiliative dimension, from disaffiliative to affiliative, or on an influence dimension, from powerful and controlling to weak and submissive. When the client's image of the other does shift, where appropriate, you can help the client elaborate and consolidate that shift by asking the client to change chairs and speak as the other: 'Tell (client) more about what life was like for you'.

Changes in self-experience. Regardless of the type of resolution attained, assisting clients to imagine and interact with the hurtful other in the empty chair creates opportunities for clients to make changes not only in how they experience the other, but also in themselves. These changes can include a shift from weak and vulnerable to strong enough to take care of self and cope with the suffering that derived from the hurtfulness, or from enraged impotence to a grounded and self-respecting assertion of boundaries. With shifts like these, clients are helped to experience themselves as free to choose how best to respond to the other and as capable of taking responsibility for those choices, independent of what the other does. Similarly, clients may shift from feeling lonely and unloved to feeling cared for and comforted. As clients' experiences of themselves shift and become more adaptive, their view of the hurtful other will also shift. For example, a person who, as a child, might have believed a harshly critical parent's assertions that they were only pointing out flaws and shortcomings because they loved the child and wanted her to do well, might as an adult client come to understand that the parent was unable or unwilling to value the client in her own right and was therefore truly insensitive and invalidating. A shift like this could enable the client to stop blaming self and set about the work of separating her own goals from the parent's goals for her.

Dealing with difficulties in letting go. If the client, speaking as the other, does not soften but instead remains critical, it's best for the counsellor to suggest that the client immediately returns to the self chair. At this point, sometimes based on what you know about the client and their story, you will have a feeling that the client wants to soften but is holding back. If that's the case, you can have the client, as self, make one more attempt to elaborate their expression of feelings and needs in order to see if a shift in the other is possible. If it then appears that no shift in the other is possible, it can be useful to ask, in a compassionate manner, 'Will you, (client's name), go to your grave still wanting this?' You can then offer an empathic formulation of the client's dilemma, for example, 'I hear that you so deeply want his/her love/approval, but at the same time you know that it will never come. I can imagine that this must leave you feeling so stuck. It's a real dilemma.' The strategy is to reframe the situation as a conflict split over whether to let go or not, which can then be worked on using the methods described in Chapter 6. Having explored the conflict split, the client may then be ready to go back into empty chair work in order to keep patiently reworking the problem.

In particular, we have found that when people have difficulty letting go of getting the other to meet the unmet need, deeper grieving is often needed. Here the person has to grieve the loss of the primary attachment figure in order to let go. In letting go of unmet needs, what was missed or lost thus has to be acknowledged, grieved, and relinquished. Letting go is giving up the hope or possibility that you are going to get what it is that you want. It is also giving up on trying to change the past. A sense of relief may ensue, but it is bittersweet.

Hanging on to the negative other provides security because it is all one had and is what one understands love to be. The person may feel that they will shatter if they let go of the unmet need. This desperate fear of annihilation must be recognized as such, and all the things the client does to avoid that anxiety must also be brought to light. Helping the client to articulate and explore such a deep yearning ('If mommy is not there, then I'll die!') can help to make more meaning out of the experience and get past old, stuck feelings of desperation. At this point you can encourage the client to do some meaning creation work (Clarke, 1989), including identifying the cherished beliefs (for example, 'If you love someone, you don't hurt them') at stake if they let go of the unmet need. This also helps with emotion regulation, as does compassionate self-soothing (described in Chapter 8). This helps the client to consider whether they can still afford to hold onto the cherished belief of getting their need met and what they might do instead (for example, 'What do I need in order to survive giving this up?'). Finally, concretizing the loss may make the grieving less overwhelming: 'Say good-bye to the things you are going to miss', 'What do these things do for you?' This is complemented with, 'How can you integrate the positive and take it with you?' or 'How can you do it for yourself?' (which takes us back to compassionate self-soothing; see Chapter 8).

Returning to Jonah, after the empty chair work in session 12, we have to peek ahead to later sessions to see what the letting go stage looked like for him: in fact, an important goal in therapy for him became to grieve not having had the mother he would have liked. In session 14, his view of his mother changed from someone who deliberately hurt him to someone who might not have been aware of hurting him, and his view of himself became that of someone whose scars were healing. Over the sessions, Jonah increased his awareness of his painful, feared emotions and was better able to tolerate them, as he assimilated some of his nonverbal emotional meaning into newly conscious formulations about himself. He became more self-accepting, reporting, 'I'm not getting down on myself as much as I used to. If I'm in a bad mood, I can say to myself, "OK, so you're in a bad mood; it won't last forever". I'm not a bad person for being in a bad mood: I'm just in a bad mood, so I'll remove myself from the situation.' In other words, Jonah no longer believed he was a bad person:

Jonah:	Anyway, the point I was trying to make here: I grew up believing that, ah, probably this is the foundation of the universe for me, that the reason, ah, my mother was always angry was because she's always mad at me, and why is she always mad at me is because I'm a bad person and you know, lower levels down.
Margaret:	That's the root of it? [empathic conjecture]
Jonah:	Yeah, I was the reason, so I, so I always, so you know from that point on, when anybody was angry, it was, I must have done something wrong.
Margaret:	Makes sense to you now. [empathic reflection]
Jonah:	Yeah, as I say, I'm trying to take a couple steps back from that and keep backing up so that I don't believe it's my fault. I won't say it doesn't happen; it does still, but it's not as violent as it used to be, and I think violent for me is a good word for how I felt about myself.

Stage 6. Post-chair work processing. When empty chair work is finished, either because the client has let go of their unresolved feelings and needs, or, more likely, because they have run out of time in the session, it's good practice for the counsellor to be ready to help the client to bring the work to a close for the moment. This can be done by commenting on the importance or challenging nature of the work and noting that you will need to end in a few minutes. If the client has at least partially resolved the task, it can be useful to take a few minutes to help them appreciate the shift they have experienced, along with any feelings of self-affirmation or empowerment. Meaning making is particularly important at the end of an intervention. You can get the client's perspective on the meaning they are making of the experience they have had in the empty chair work; this helps them build this into a shared formulation of how their process works, including key stuck points and directions forward. This also helps to consolidate post-session gains. However, it is important not to start with meaning making too early. It needs to come *after* the client has experienced emotional arousal; otherwise, it risks becoming empty conceptualizing, which won't change anything. This emphasis on making meaning on the basis of aroused emotional experience is what distinguishes EFT from more purely interpretative and cognitive approaches. In addition, awareness homework may be offered after sessions of empty chair work, to highlight discoveries already made in the session. For example, 'During the week, see if you can pay attention to times when your anger collapses into sadness'. Or for a client who is blocked by self-interruption, you can have them notice how they stop themselves from feeling emotions. It's even OK to suggest that clients keep a diary. For example, you can suggest that they sit down

each evening to list at least three emotions they felt that day, or what they are feeling towards the other, and so on.

Going back to Jonah's session 12, the session ended with Jonah acknowledging that his problem is rage:

Jonah:	But then when I do try and stand up, I mean, I get this huge rage and I'm on the edge of snapping.
Margaret:	That rage is what we need to tap into here. Because there's a lot of rage, not surprisingly. [empathic formulation]
Jonah:	But what's the point? That I'm not- (sigh) How do you mean tap into it?
Margaret:	Well, deal with your anger.
Jonah:	That won't solve anything, will it?
Margaret:	Mm-hm (pause) mm-hm. It won't change your mom, it won't change your boss, but it can change you if you get its message and see what needs to be done about it. You're walking around with a powder keg inside of you (pause) and, things trigger it, all the time. But underneath the anger I think is the terrible fear and shame. [empathic formulation of client process]
Jonah:	Mm, (sigh) I never thought of myself as angry.
Margaret:	Yeah, well, just think about it, and see, I don't mean going around suddenly expressing the anger, but just give it some thought over the next week, and, pay attention to how often you actually feel frustration or anger. [awareness homework]
Jonah:	I just never really thought I was angry at my mother. I thought it was the other-, all the other shit that goes on a daily basis (sniff).
Margaret:	So now it's occurring to you that you have a fair bit of anger at your mom as well. [process reflection]
Jonah:	And not just for current or future behaviour.
Margaret:	No, because of the hurt from the past as well.
Jonah:	I guess I'm angry that she doesn't acknowledge it.

Variations in Empty Chair Work

As you can see, empty chair work is a large and complex task, rich with possibilities and nuances that will take quite a bit of focused practice to master. In this section we touch on some of the variations of empty chair work, including trauma-focused empty chair work, current conflictual relationships, and speaking your truth, an alternative to empty chair work.

Empty chair work with trauma. It is important to note that pushing the client to do empty chair work is unwise and possibly harmful under two sets of circumstances: first, when the unresolved experience was severely traumatizing and there is a risk of re-traumatization; and second, when the client has a recent history of behaviours that are self-harming (for example, self-mutilation or suicide attempts) or other-harming (for example, aggressive and violent acting-out behaviours, or impulsive risk-taking that puts others in danger). When such behaviours have become part of the way the client responds to intense distress or arousal, it is strongly recommended that the counsellor uses less evocative interventions, at least initially, delaying the introduction of interventions like empty chair work until after a strong therapeutic relationship is well established, and a set of adaptive emotion moderation strategies have been established. (See Table 3.2; e.g., identifying a safe place that the client can go to internally). Establishing sufficient internal and external support to face an imagined abusive other is essential before introducing empty chair dialogue.

Trauma-based empty chair work is typically more intense than when the unfinished business is related to neglect or poor parenting. In trauma-based injury, the person is fragile (easily emotionally dysregulated) and suffers from unwanted memories and debilitating emotional pain. To promote enduring change, it is important to attend to and help the person first develop ways of dealing with the dysregulated emotion. People with this type of problem, however, are often ambivalent about whether or not they want to return to face the source of the trauma, which includes engaging in empty chair work with abusers. On the one hand, they are drawn to the issue in an attempt to rid themselves of the intrusive memories. On the other hand, there is significant pain that threatens to dysregulate and re-traumatize the person. As a result, empty chair work should only be suggested when safety has been established and the clients feel ready to face their abusers (Paivio & Pascual-Leone, 2010).

In working through emotional injuries in abusive relationships, empty chair work is used to help the client to express anger to the abusive other within the safety of the session. This helps the client to make more effective boundaries with the other. In contrast, however, it is generally better not to express sadness to the abusive other. Each emotion needs to find its appropriate object, and so sadness may need to be expressed to the counsellor or to someone else in the person's life, such as a protective other, rather than to the abusive other.

In situations of past abuse and terrorization, the core fear felt in the original situations often remains coded at a body level, where it is difficult to work with. This trauma-related fear needs to be countered with adaptive anger. As long as the anger remains buried beneath the fear, the person can protest forever but will not improve and will continue to feel helpless. What is needed for transformation is a mobilization of the protective adaptive anger that could not be expressed in the original situation. People who have been trapped in traumatic experiences have been unable to perform any of the actions they needed to save themselves. What is needed is promotion of the action tendencies and the ultimate feeling of triumph over oppression. The person needs to experience themselves as able to vanquish the perpetrator in order to overcome the feeling of being vanquished. The anger needs to be directed outwards rather than towards the self, and to be differentiated from the other emotions (for example, sadness, shame or pain), so it is clearly felt and the client can use the action tendency to set a boundary. In addition, the anger needs to be expressed assertively with a full sense of agency and ownership rather than as a victim, and at a level of intensity appropriate to the situation. Finally, the meaning embodied in the anger needs to be explored, symbolized and elaborated, so that it can become a resource for the person.

Variant marker/task: Current conflictual relationship. We said at the beginning of this chapter that empty chair work is best carried out with past emotional injuries. There is, however, a variant form of the marker: *current interpersonal conflict*, in which the person is currently struggling with someone in their environment. If, for example, there is current spousal conflict about childrearing practices or ongoing physical or emotional abuse, empty chair work needs to be done differently and has somewhat different goals, because of the risk that the client will use the task as a rehearsal for strong expression of feelings, which may very well be counter-productive in their current situation. There are, however, mixed situations where a current interpersonal difficulty evokes unfinished business: for instance, a young adult client who is having some current difficulty with his mother, whom he complains nags him about not keeping his room tidy or washing the dishes (current situation), but also experiences her behaviour and attitude as evoking what has been happening since the death of his father when the client was nine years old (for example, 'Ever since he passed she has expected me to be her support'). He is in a current interpersonal conflict but also has unfinished business. Unfinished business from the past differs from current interpersonal conflict. In helping a client with a current conflictual situation, the goal is clarification of what is truly felt (primary adaptive emotions) and then a focus on what the client needs to do based on what is felt. In standard unfinished business, the purpose is to process unresolved past feelings and the goal is not how to handle the person in the present but to resolve painful stuck emotion.

Speaking your truth: An alternative to empty chair work. It is also possible to work on the process of resolving past emotional injury without actually having the person speak to an empty chair. You can facilitate the resolution process described above (and in Table 7.1) by empathically following and guiding without enactment. This can be done using a focusing process (see Chapter 5). You can say such things as 'What would you say to them if they were here?', 'If you could speak your truth about them, what would you say to them?' You can even work with the other's imagined response: 'What do you imagine they would say back?', 'What kinds of things did they say to you in the past?', and 'Imagine hearing that. What does that feel like?' Imagery can also be used in a variety of other ways to evoke the unresolved emotion. The visual system is highly related to emotion, so imagination can be used to create a kind of theatre of the mind: to evoke an unresolved emotion, to enact dialogues in imagination, to experience new emotions, or to imagine adding people or resources to situations or scenes to help the client experience the scene in a new way.

A short outline of this alternative is given below:

- **Establish contact**: Ask the client to imagine the other in their mind.
- **Access the feeling**: Ask the client 'What do you feel in your body?' (e.g., C: 'I feel heavy, sad.')
    - Help the client sink into this experience and taste it by asking them where in their body they feel this and inviting them to stay with the feeling (e.g., C: 'I feel it in my chest. Here. And I felt so alone.')

- Ask the client 'What did you miss?'. This intervention helps unpack sadness and open it out with a suggestion such as 'Imagine telling them what it's like, what you missed'.
- Validate the hurt (even if you hear anger in the background).

- **Access the need in the feeling**: Ask the client 'Imagine telling them what you needed' (e.g., C: 'I just needed you to tell me you loved me.')
- **Adaptive emotion often emerges**: Offer empathic affirmation to the suffering and anguish; move into the compassionate self-soothing task (see Chapter 8).

Further Exploration

Reading

Elliott, R., Watson, J.C., Goldman, R. N., Greenberg, L. S. (2004). *Learning emotion-focused therapy: The process-experiential approach to change.* Washington, DC: American Psychological Association. [Chapter 12]

Greenberg, L. S., & Woldarsky Meneses, C. (2019). *Forgiveness and letting go in emotion-focused therapy.* Washington, DC: American Psychological Association. [Chapters 3 and 4]

Watching

Elliott, R. (2016). *Understanding Emotion-Focused Therapy with Robert Elliott.* Counselling Channel Videos, Glastonbury, UK. Available at: https://vimeo.com/ondemand/understandingeft/167235549 [Inexpensive demonstration session with male client featuring empty chair work and compassionate self-soothing]

Greenberg, L. S. (2007). *Emotion-Focused Therapy for depression.* American Psychological Association Videos. [See session 2 of this two-session video for clear example of empty chair work]

Reflecting

1. There is a lot of information in this chapter. (It's the longest chapter in this book.) If you've finished reading through it, take a minute to consider the following questions:

   - What was your experience of reading it?
   - Thinking back over what you've read in this chapter, see if you can remember three points that you found useful or interesting. Make a note of these.

2. This chapter has a lot of transcript of Jonah's counselling in it. Ask a friend or colleague to go through the different sections, enacting the roles of Jonah and his counsellor Margaret. (This is one form of *deliberate practice* and can be useful for beginning to learn a new approach to counselling.)

3. Using your own personal experience, identify an unresolved issue with someone who has been important in your life, someone who has shaped who you are, for better or worse. (This could be a parent, sibling, best friend or partner, or important authority figure, such as a teacher or boss.) Write a brief description of what's unresolved. Then, on your own, without anyone else around, imagine them present, perhaps in another chair, and try telling them about the issue. Pay attention to what it feels like to do this.

8

Late Working Phase: Empathic Affirmation and Compassionate Self-Soothing

---

Chapter Outline

Working with Vulnerability and Emotional Pain

Empathic Affirmation for Vulnerability: A Classic Person-Centred Task

Compassionate Self-Soothing for Anguish

Bethany's Late Working Phase

Further Exploration

Working with Vulnerability and Emotional Pain

Client vulnerability, strong emotional pain and anguish are a common occurrence in the late working phase of EFC. In this chapter we present two related tasks. The common thread in these markers is painful vulnerability. These tasks emerge increasingly as the working phase of EFC progresses and the client moves towards their core pain. The first of these, *Empathic Affirmation for Vulnerability*, comes out of the person–centred tradition and was mapped by Laura Rice and Les Greenberg (Rice & Greenberg, 1991); the second, *Compassionate Self-Soothing for Anguish*, became prominent within EFC in the 2000s (Goldman & Fox, 2010; Ito, Greenberg, Iwakabe, & Pascual-Leone, 2010; Sutherland, Peräkylä & Elliott, 2014), especially as EFC began to be applied to anxiety difficulties. These two tasks complement each other. Vulnerability is primarily a here-and-now feeling, for example, 'I have no skin, so exposed and unprotected'. On the other hand, anguish is more related to evoked past memories of the emotional suffering of feeling vulnerable and without support, often from childhood experiences. Vulnerability occurring in relation to present circumstances is best worked with in the client–counsellor relationship, while anguish generally is best worked with using chair work, in an extension of two chair and empty chair work. Because both involve vulnerability, they can sometimes be used as alternatives to each other, for example, when the client refuses chair work or when therapist empathic affirmation is not enough to help the client move forward.

Empathic Affirmation for Vulnerability: A Classic Person-Centred Task

Person-centred counselling has a rich body of practice, and it was from this that Laura Rice, one of the founders of EFC, drew in formulating Empathic Affirmation for Vulnerability. In this task, the work is carried entirely within the client–counsellor dialogue. While EFC tasks in general seek to combine doing and being, in Empathic Affirmation the emphasis is very much on the side of *being*. The counsellor attempts to stay strongly empathically connected and present while the client plumbs the depths of their vulnerability and gets to their core pain. Table 8.1 lays out this classic person-centred task, in which the counsellor provides strong empathy, compassion and validation to the client. As the task progresses, the counsellor also pays close attention to any signs from the client that they are beginning to access hope or growth, or even just allowing self to feel understood, validated or comforted/soothed.

TABLE 8.1 *Empathic affirmation for vulnerability: Task resolution model*

Task Resolution Stage	Counsellor Responses
1. *Marker: Intense Vulnerability*. Expresses strong negative self-related distress (e.g., fragility, shame, despair, hopelessness, exhaustion), primarily based in the present.	• Listen for, reflect vulnerability. • Allow self to resonate with client's emotional pain, access genuine compassion for client.
2. *Initial Deepening*. Describes form of vulnerability, allows deeper feelings to emerge in response to counsellor's empathic affirmation.	• Switch to Empathic Affirmation/Prizing: • Empathic understanding, dwelling on form of vulnerability. • Slow, gentle manner. • Offer empathic validation, support client self-soothing as needed.
3. *Intense Deepening/Touching Bottom*. Expresses dreaded emotion or painful aspect of self in full intensity; seems to touch bottom.	• Continue Empathic Affirmation/Prizing mode. • Listen for, offer metaphors to capture, deepen vulnerability.

Task Resolution Stage	Counsellor Responses
4. **Turning Back up towards Growth/ Hope**. Expresses needs/action tendencies associated with primary adaptive emotions.	• Listen for, reflect, dwell on hope/growth needs or action tendencies.
5. **Appreciating**. Describes or expresses reduced distress, greater calmness; expresses appreciation of connection to counsellor; expresses sense of self as whole, acceptable or capable.	• Explore, support sense of relief, calm. • Explore, support changes in self-scheme.
6. **Processing**. Emerges out of the vulnerable state. Reflects on the work, creates meaning.	• Help client to reflect on the work and its meaning.

*The vulnerability marker.*Vulnerability is a particular form of emotional pain in which the person feels fragile, deeply ashamed or insecure in the present moment in their life: 'I just feel like I've got nothing left. I'm finished. It's too much to ask of myself to carry on.' Vulnerability is a state of current weakness and fragility in the face of life's stresses. It can take different forms, including more emergent, primary adaptive pain brought into awareness by in-session exploration, but also more general, stuck (primary maladaptive) vulnerability that is present in a person's current situation, which they are bringing into therapy as a problematic state to be dealt with. In these states of vulnerability people feel deeply vulnerable, like they have no skin to protect themselves, and they may feel secondary shame or insecurity about their vulnerability. Clients in these states need, above all else, solid empathic attunement from the counsellor, who must not only capture the content of what the client is feeling, but also note the energy and emotions of the client, mirroring the tempo, rhythm, and tone of the experience. In addition, it's useful for the counsellor to validate and normalize the client's experience. Resolution involves accessing resilience and the will to carry on, and results in a strengthened sense of self. One of our favourite examples of this task is Carl Rogers' 1955 film, Miss Mun (quoted in Greenberg et al., 1993; see also Gundrum, Lietaer, & Hees-Matthijssen, 1999), a brief excerpt of which we give here:

Miss Mun [hesitantly]:	And I'm frightened, because I kind of feel that they're having to be sure that it isn't cancer. And that really frightens me (Rogers: Mhm) terribly, and, I think it's when I've let that thought come to me: 'Maybe it is and what if it is', that's when I felt so *dreadfully* alone [= vulnerability marker]
Rogers:	Mhm. Then, if it's *really* something like that, then you must feel, *so* alone. [empathic affirmation response]
Miss Mun:	(pause) And it's really a frightening kind of loneliness, because I don't know who could be with you.
Rogers:	Is this what you're saying? Could *anyone* be with you in, in, fear, or in loneliness like that?

Miss Mun:	(weeping during a long pause)
Rogers:	It just really cuts *so* deep. [empathic affirmation, also evocative reflection]

The main challenges for the counsellor in this task are allowing self to deeply resonate with the client's intense vulnerability in order to access genuine compassion for them; and then having faith that if the client is able to go deep enough into the pain, they will hit bottom (reach core pain) and then spontaneously turn back up towards hope and forward movement out of their stuckness, as illustrated by the following exchange a bit later from Miss Mun's session with Rogers:

Miss Mun:	(long pause). I guess probably *basically* there'd be a part of it you *would* have to do alone. I, I mean you just couldn't maybe take anyone else along in some of the feeling. And yet, it would be sort of a comfort, I guess, not to be alone.
Rogers:	It surely would be nice if you could take someone with you a good deal of the way into your, feelings of aloneness, and fear.
Miss Mun:	(pause). I guess I just *have.*

We want to point out here that it's important for the counsellor not to rush in to try to fix, over-regulate or over-validate the client in their distress, but instead to be patient and allow time for the client to receive and take in the counsellor's empathic affirmation, thus beginning the process of translating counsellor affirmation into self-affirmation. More information about this task can be found in Elliott et al. (2004) and Greenberg et al. (1993).

Compassionate Self-Soothing for Anguish

The other, more recent EFC task for working with client anguish is a form of two chair work in which the client enacts comforting or soothing self. This is essentially the opposite of two chair self-critical split work (described in Chapter 6); at the same time, this work often emerges in the last stages of empty chair work, when the client confronts the fact that the person who they hoped would satisfy their unmet need will never be able to do so.

There are of course many maladaptive kinds of self-soothing, in which we attempt to block out, numb or distract from uncomfortable or painful feelings, for example by using substances or engaging in risky, impulsive activities. These simply cover up or delay the discomfort, leaving the underlying pain unattended to, and often make it worse. In general, emotional suffering (regardless of whether we call it vulnerability or anguish) occurs in the face of powerful unmet interpersonal needs (e.g., for love or validation) left over from our history and made worse by our negative self-treatment. These needs have to be addressed in order for the pain to be eased.

The anguish marker. Anguish, a more general marker than vulnerability, is evoked from memories in which one, often as a child, was unsupported, neglected, left painfully alone or invalidated. It refers to strong emotional pain, which can take a variety of forms, and can be under-regulated and disorganizing, or over-regulated and at least partially interrupted. It is clearest when the client is suffering emotionally, and feels terribly alone and unsupported, based on a history of abandonment or humiliation. This is often the case in people who commit self-harm or use self-medication to regulate their emotions. When the anguish is experienced as a kind of emotional wound or injury from having one's basic needs ignored or trampled on, either by others or by self, it is particularly appropriate as a marker for the compassionate self-soothing task.

The task. Compassion is the opposite of self-criticism; expressing compassion towards oneself is a way of changing painful emotions (e.g., shame, fear, sadness) by internally confronting a painful feeling with a different emotion. The work of compassionate self-soothing involves helping the client imagine or enact a comforting, affirming person who can give an anguished self what it needs, often re-entering a scene of deprivation or invalidation and offering compassion and some sort of self-soothing or self-comforting where none was available before. This can be done in various ways, depending on what is being worked on and what most fits for the client; see Table 8.2 for an outline of the different options.

TABLE 8.2 *Dimensions of compassionate self-soothing*

1. Modes (how soothing/comfort is carried out):
   a. Guided Imagination
   b. Dialogue Enactment

2. Sources/Resources (who provides the soothing/comfort):
   a. Adult/current self
   b. Real or imagined caring parental figure

3. Objects (who receives the soothing/comfort):
   a. Current vulnerable self
   b. Child self
   c. Other child (specific or universal)
   d. Other vulnerable being (e.g., similar friend or pet)

4. Forms (response modes):
   a. Showing empathy ('It's a hard way to live your life.')
   b. Disclosing caring/love ('I love you.')
   c. Praising/validating ('You are good at this.')
   d. Offering caring advice ('You need to be the best you can and that's all anybody asks.')
   e. Offering protection ('I'll keep you safe; I won't let them hurt you anymore.')
   f. Providing company ('I'm right here; I'm not going anywhere.')

For example, if the anguish marker has emerged out of empty chair work, a useful approach is to propose that the client imagines the client's adult self re-entering an evoked scene and providing a caring response to their lost/lonely/wounded child self; or this can be done as a dialogue between chairs, in which the client is asked to speak from one chair as their adult self, to soothe their wounded child in the other chair. The goal here is to evoke compassion for the self. Self-compassion and self-empathy can be developed from the client internalizing these qualities from a compassionate, empathic counsellor (as in the Empathic Affirmation task described earlier); however, this internalization can take many sessions of therapy. Suggesting that the client as an adult offers compassion to the suffering self in the session can speed up and facilitate this process.

Table 8.3 summarizes this task.

TABLE 8.3   *Compassionate self-soothing for emotional suffering or anguish: Task resolution model*

Client Resolution Stages	Counsellor Facilitating Responses
1. *Marker*: Expressing anguish (unregulated shame/fear or unmet existential needs) with familiar despair and stuckness, partially symbolized and primarily based on past experiences.	Reflect marker; propose task
2. *Entering*: Identifying and beginning role play of appropriate form of Experiencing Self and Compassionate Other.	• Propose or help client to identify an appropriate self–other combination to enact; adapt as needed. • Ask client to imagine the Experiencing Self and Compassionate Other; use evocative language. • Provide solid empathy for client anguish and familiar despair and stuckness.
3. *Deepening*: Protesting/grieving that compassion/self-soothing are impossible; confronting existential nature of absent soothing.	• Propose self-soothing of Experiencing Self by Compassionate Other. • Validate protest and confrontation with perceived impossibility of being soothed. • Support client in holding non-supportive others accountable. • Help client to enter confrontation by making it clear that although they may not have known this previously, they now have the option to offer support/compassion to themselves. • Help client to access primary emotion and what it longs for/needs/might help. • Offer strong therapeutic presence.
4. *Partial resolution*: Offering self-soothing.	• Listen for, reflect bodily felt shift in response to compassionate, soothing offer. • Encourage client to stay with the new feeling.
5. Experiencing emotional/bodily relief; shifting towards more positive, empowered sense of self.	• Help client to explore the emergent, stronger sense of self. • Validate more empowered sense of self.
6. *Full resolution:* Considering how to extend this process in their life.	• Help client explore possibilities for carrying self-soothing or empowered self forward in their life.

As an example, the counsellor can ask the client to imagine a child sitting in a chair in front of him or her, a child who has suffered what that person has suffered in life. To evoke the child's plight the counsellor next describes the most poignant details of the person's history and then asks, 'What would you say to that child? What do you feel towards the child?' This typically evokes a compassionate response towards the child and the child's circumstances and a recognition of what the child needed. Here is an example of a female counsellor we'll call Zahra working with a female client named Nour:

Zahra:	Imagine an 8-year-old sitting there. Her mother hardly looks at her, never mind talks to her. Her father emotionally draws on her for all the love he can't get from his wife and then rejects her when he doesn't need her. What do you imagine it's like for her?
Nour:	I don't know. She just feels so bad about herself.
Zahra:	What would you say to her if she were your child?
Nour:	I know she would feel so alone without anyone. She deserves more.
Zahra:	Can you give her some of what she needs?
Nour:	I see you, and I want you to know that you are not alone; I'm here.
Zahra:	Now, can you imagine the sad, lonely child part of you in the chair there?
Nour:	Yeah, OK.
Zahra:	Can you respond to her in the same way? Let her know she's not alone. What else can you say to her?

Suggestions for facilitating compassionate self-soothing. In this task, it often seems important to start with a stranger or a child in general, not with the part of the self that needs soothing. Even though people understand the implication of what they are being asked to do, they seem to be better able to soothe a child in general. Once the softening has occurred in relation to a child in need, it is easier to transfer this feeling to the self. Over time, doing this in conjunction with the empathic affirmation provided by the counsellor's affective attunement helps the person develop their self-soothing capacity.

In this task, the counsellor first helps the client to deepen their sense of anguish so that they can access their core pain and the unmet needs associated with it. Then, the counsellor can offer a two chair process, described above, in which the client is asked to enact providing what is needed (e.g., validation, support, protection) to themselves. The source of comforting is represented either as a strong, nurturing aspect of self or as an idealized parental figure or some other positive force. Resolution in this task involves not only feeling compassion for self, but accessing the unmet need and grieving that was never met and feeling compassion for what was lost.

Imagery also can be used in a variety of other ways to evoke emotion in this task. The visual system is closely related to emotion, so imagination can be used to evoke an unresolved emotion, to enact dialogues in imagination to experience a new emotion, or to imagine adding people or resources to situations or scenes to help one experience the scene in a new way. Thus, one can ask the client to imagine re-entering a scene or a time of their life to access their core pain and can facilitate transforming the painful emotion by expressing what was needed or by bringing a protector into a childhood scene. The protector can offer the protection that was missing or have them imagine bringing in resources that will empower or protect the person, like a lock and key to secure their room, or a cage in which to put the feared person. This helps generate a new emotion to change the old emotion. For example, the counsellor might say:

Try closing your eyes and remembering the experience of yourself in a situation. Get a concrete image if you can. Go into it. Be your child in this scene. Please tell me what is happening. What do you see, smell, hear in the situation? What do you feel in your body and what is going through your mind?

After a while the counsellor can ask the client to shift perspectives by saying:

Now I would like you to view the scene as an adult now. What do you see, feel and think? Do you see the look on the child's face? What do you want to do? Do it. How can you intervene? Try it now in imagination.

Changing perspectives again, the counsellor can ask the client to become the child:

What as the child do you feel and think? What do you need from the adult? Ask for what you need or wish for. What does the adult do? What else do you need? Ask for it. Is there someone else you would like to come in to help? Receive the care and protection offered.

This intervention concludes with the counsellor helping the client to process the experience, for example by asking:

Check how you feel now. What does all this mean, to you about you, and about what you needed? Come back to the present, to yourself as an adult now. How do you feel? Can you say goodbye to the child for now?

Bethany's Late Working Phase

The late working phase of Bethany's counselling, especially from session 9 to 15, illustrates the key role played by the empty chair work and compassionate self-soothing and how these build on focusing and two chair work from the early working phase of EFC, with a supporting role played by Empathic Affirmation. In session 6 Bethany has her initial experience of empty chair work with her mother, who dismisses Bethany's apology for having been an angry teenager; Robert then suggests that she puts her father in the other chair, and it turns out that he is much more supportive and caring.

Bethany's session 9 illustrates much of we've covered in Chapters 7 and 8. Part way through the session she reveals that she feels like crying but is stopping herself by calling herself stupid; they move briefly into two chair work on this self-interruption split, and she realizes that she is terrified of crying. The counsellor asks her what she is so scared of, and she remembers that when she was a small child her mother scolded her for crying, which he initially meets by providing empathic affirmation responses. They then move into Empty Chair Work with Bethany's mother, and the counsellor has Bethany move over to the other chair and enact her mother telling her off: 'Don't be so pathetic, stop crying, grow up.' As herself, Bethany reports feeling first scared and then sad and lonely. With help from the counsellor she reconstructs and re-experiences the whole process: her mother looks 'angry and sharp'; then Bethany gets scared of being hurt and starts to cry. She remembers her mother's look of contempt and the tone of her voice, how she felt ashamed, then sad/lonely, then finally ran off to her friend's family. Moving into a Compassionate Self-Soothing task, the counsellor suggests that she be the sad, lonely, ashamed little girl, and asks, 'What does that little girl need?' Bethany says, 'Emotional freedom'. Remembering her much more positive relation with her father, the counsellor then proposes, 'Change this, face her, put little Bethany there. Be your dad, what could you give her?' Crying, she says, 'Don't be scared of your feelings, whatever you feel. I want you to be comfortable to be yourself. Just embrace how you feel.' The counsellor then has Bethany come back over to the self chair, and asks her, 'Can you let that in?' However, she is unable to do this, so the counsellor suggests instead that Bethany imagines her 1-year-old daughter in the other chair. After a pause, she says she really wants her daughter to have that freedom. The counsellor asks her, 'Who could give Bethany that freedom?' The client replies, 'Myself'. The counsellor then asks her, 'Be the voice that says it's OK to be sad', and coaches her through telling herself, 'It's alright, what's the worst thing that could happen? I know you're scared, but it will be OK.' Running out of time in the session, the counsellor asks Bethany how she feels at this point, and she describes a sense of relief from the pressure she felt coming into the session today. They then move into talking about how the session has gone. She says she feels she's been in an internal battle and is exhausted but less tense in her body. After briefly reviewing the session, the counsellor proposes awareness homework ('Pay attention to what that little girl in you needs'). Bethany leaves the session feeling pleased.

In session 11, Bethany comes back to Empty Chair Work with her mother, as she re-experiences how her mother rejected her 14-year-old self as a harmful monster, and how she and her dog used to escape from the house for long walks together. Exploring her relationship with the dog, the counsellor has the client put the dog in the other chair and then provide Compassionate Self-Soothing to herself from the dog chair. In session 12, she again puts her mother in the empty chair in order to speak her deepest truths to her. After this session, without prompting from the counsellor, she tries to talk with her mother in reality, but is dissatisfied by the perfunctory thanks her mother offers. Thus, in session 13, the counsellor has Bethany offer reassurance to the let-down, disappointed part of her, from a strong, caring part of herself. There is one more piece of Compassionate Self-Soothing chair work in session 15, which we will describe in the next chapter.

Further Exploration

Reading

Elliott, R., Watson, J. C., Goldman, R. N., & Greenberg, L. S. (2004). *Learning emotion-focused therapy: The process-experiential approach to change.* Washington, DC: American Psychological Association. [See Chapter 7 for presentation of Empathic Affirmation task]

Gundrum, M., Lietaer, G., & Van Hees-Matthijssen, C. (1999). Carl Rogers' responses in the 17th session with Miss Mun: Comments from a process-experiential and psychoanalytic perspective. *British Journal of Guidance & Counselling, 27*(4), 461–482. [Complete transcript and analysis of Carl Rogers session featuring Empathic Affirmation task]

Sutherland, O., Peräkylä, A., & Elliott, R. (2014). Conversation analysis of the two-chair self-soothing task in emotion-focused therapy. *Psychotherapy Research, 24*, 738–751. doi: 10.1080/10503307.2014.885146 [Detailed analysis of the Compassionate Self-Soothing task]

Watching

Elliott, R. (2016). *Understanding Emotion-Focused Therapy with Robert Elliott.* Counselling Channel Videos, Glastonbury, UK. Available at: https://vimeo.com/ondemand/understandingeft/167235549 [Inexpensive demonstration session with male client featuring empty chair work and compassionate self-soothing]

Psychotherapy.net (2014). *Carl Rogers and the Person-Centered Approach.* Available online at: www.youtube.com/watch?v=mmgOxMsBaJI [Brief YouTube promotional video features a video clip illustrating a vulnerability marker and an example of an empathic affirmation response from Miss Mun case, the example cited in this chapter]

Reflecting

1. Questions for journaling: What is your relation to strong emotional pain in yourself or others? How do you respond when you encounter strong emotional pain? Do you find yourself deflecting away from it? What strategies do you use to deal with it? Do these strategies aim to numb the pain or distract yourself from it? In what ways would you like to be able to comfort yourself when you are hurting? What stops you?

2. See if you can find something that hurts emotionally; give yourself time to feel it. Next, ask the pain what hurts the most about it; again, give yourself time to feel this. Finally, ask this pain what it needs. See what happens and try to pay attention to any places where you get stuck in trying this.

9

Consolidation Phase: The Work of Ending Well

Chapter Outline

Overview of the Ending Process

Bethany's Consolidation Phase

Ending as a Therapeutic Task

Variations in Ending

Jonah Finishes Counselling

Further Exploration

Overview of the Ending Process

The process of ending appropriately is an essential aspect of good EFC practice. In EFC, endings of sessions are times for stepping back and reflecting on the meaning of the often-difficult emotion work that the client has been involved in. This applies to an even greater extent to the end of counselling, where client and counsellor engage in a more extended process of creating a meaning perspective and consolidating an emotionally grounded, shared story of how the client's problematic process worked and how they can continue to become more emotionally flexible and alive with self and others. Of course, we recognize that for many reasons counselling often ends before the client feels finished, and that it is important to support the client regardless of the nature of the ending, which may either occur naturally, when the client feels they have done the work they needed to do (at least for the moment), or may be to some degree limited by time or other circumstances before the client feels done. It's also true that the counsellor may have strong or unexpected feelings about ending, and in such situations it is useful for them to remain curious about these and to be ready to draw on them as appropriate.

Bethany's Consolidation Phase

The beginning of Bethany's consolidation phase. Bethany's counselling provides an example of a carefully planned and thoroughly processed ending of counselling in which the client feels ready to end. Session 15 (discussed at the end of the previous chapter) is the overlap between her late working phase and her ending phase of counselling. At the beginning of this session Robert reminds her that after today they have a maximum of five more sessions left. Beginning the process of ending, Bethany tells him that she has been worrying about this, because she has come to appreciate the value of having a safe place to talk about whatever is bothering her. She reports that for her this has been freeing and is a very new experience. She compares herself to a polar bear raised in a zoo. Now, she says, she has raised her 'benchmark' of what she wants and needs from herself and others, and is hoping to be able to develop more openness with her husband; she sees him as very much up for this.

Towards the end of this session, Bethany reflects that before counselling she experienced her anxiety as coming from inside her. At this point the counsellor offers what we have found to be a sometimes-helpful method of using a visual formulation of how her difficult process works. With her agreement he pulls out a piece of paper and with her help he draws a flow chart of their shared understanding of it, working backwards from her social anxiety to her primary maladaptive guilt/shame at being damaging. Her core pain is devastation (in her words: 'I have ruined everything') and leaves her feeling utterly alone and abandoned. Client and counsellor review what this sense of devastation needs: 'protection, affirmation; to belong to the family and be wanted'. Building on this formulation, Bethany then does another piece of validating self-soothing work, speaking from her adult self to her 14 year-old self: 'It's not your fault; you were doing the best you knew how to do', and she is finally able to begin to let this in. Processing this session, the counsellor offers Bethany the drawing they made of her process, and suggests that their work for the remaining sessions could be about the process of helping her build what she calls 'resilience'.

Final sessions. In session 16, Bethany applies the work she has been doing on herself to two currently challenging interpersonal situations, and is able to stand up to the critical/coercive part of herself without falling into anxiety about ruining relationships and damaging others. In session 17, Bethany looks back over her counselling and appreciates how far she has come. Halfway through, the counsellor asks Bethany how she is now with her social anxiety about being damaging to other people; she replies that she is far less worried about this now. In response to her wish for further practice with self-soothing, they do a bit more work of this, which makes it clear that she has eased up on herself in difficult interpersonal situations. She then reports that she understands what was involved in her fear of other people, where it came from, and has largely resolved the issue. Nevertheless, she notes that being afraid of other people is a kind of 'habit of thought' that is taking time to diminish. The counsellor normalizes this, agreeing that it does take time, and they agree to space out their final three sessions.

In session 18, after working on a minor current conflictual relationship, client and counsellor move into processing their experiences of the counselling. Bethany says that she does feel ready to end counselling, but has decided she wants one more session; they agree to meet again, in five weeks. Robert shares his appreciation of how hard she has worked and how far she has come; she says appreciatively. 'We've *both* worked really hard!' Then five weeks later, at the beginning of session 19, Bethany confirms that she still feels ready to end and that this will be their last session. She reports that she has handled the previous five weeks without difficulty and has in fact been practising being herself with other people 'who are lot more risky than you are'. Near the end of the session she reports that she feels pleased, proud of how far she has come, while also a bit sad about ending. She discloses that the counselling has been very important for her, tearing up as she says this; the counsellor tears up also. Bethany reports that she now feels ready 'to be an adult'; the counsellor shares his experience of having learned from her and how he will carry a sense of her with him.

Ending as a Therapeutic Task

The case of Bethany illustrates several aspects of the process of ending in EFC. A key point is for counsellors to be attuned to the range of different emotions that ending counselling is likely to raise for clients, especially sadness, but also anxiety and pride (cf. Greenberg, 2002). The first general principle is to be as curious as always, because every client will have their own unique experience of ending therapy; our clients continue to surprise us in how they respond in ending.

A second general principle is to think of ending counselling as a therapeutic task, with a series of stages to it. Table 9.1 provides a model of ending work in EFC, using the six-stage format we've offered for other therapeutic tasks; most of these steps are clearly exemplified in the consolidation/ending phase of Bethany's counselling.

TABLE 9.1 *Ending work: Subtasks and therapist facilitative work of therapy termination*

Subtask	Therapist Facilitative Work
1. *Marker*: Impending end of counselling.	• Recognize when it's time to start preparing the client to end.
2. *Preparing the way*: Preparing client for ending.	• Clarify and remind client about time limits from the beginning of counselling. • Allow 3–4 sessions at end for unresolved issues. • Suggest reserving time for ending work. • Allow time between sessions for personal reflection on (a) how client is likely to experience ending and (b) how counsellor feels about the ending.

(Continued)

TABLE 9.1 *(Continued)*

Subtask	Therapist Facilitative Work
3. *Exploring client's experience of ending.*	• Empathic Exploration of hopes and fears about ending. • Set aside assumptions about client's experience of ending.
4. *Looking ahead*: Exploring continuing and future life projects.	• Empathic Exploration of what is next for them following the end of counselling.
5. *Doing the ending*: ○ Exploring client's experience of progress (or lack of it). ○ Mutual sharing of experience of therapy.	• Help client to explore 'then–now' contrast from before to after counselling. • Personal reassurance/normalizing about client's state/progress (as appropriate and genuine). • Self-disclosure of own genuine reaction to ending.
6. *Post-ending reflection*: ○ Client and counsellor reflect on their work together and what they are taking away from it.	• Client: Can be contacted at a later date to collect follow-up data or reflections. • Counsellor: Can use personal supervision or journaling to reflect on what they've learned or to address any unresolved issues they are left with.

1. Impending end marker. The marker of this task is of course the impending end of counselling, indicated by a sense that because of the dwindling number of sessions it is now time to start tying the work up rather than opening new, deep or painful issues. This will vary with things like the overall length of counselling, whether it is open-ended versus time-limited, how emotionally fragile the client is, how successful counselling has been, and whether the work is coming to a natural end or is still ongoing. Longer-term or open-ended counselling and work with more fragile clients and with less success and still ongoing issues all require more time and effort to be put into the ending process. On the other hand, if there is a six-session limit, you'll want to remind the client from the beginning about the time limit, but you'll only be able to devote one or at most two sessions to the process of ending. In contrast, if you've got up to 20 sessions, it can be very useful to devote three to five sessions to the ending process, as illustrated by Bethany's counselling, in order to help the client consolidate the progress they've made.

2. Preparing the way. In the first place, it's important that time limits are made clear from the beginning of counselling. If the number of sessions allowed is 10 to 20 sessions, the counsellor can remind the client of this every few sessions. The attitude is that the counsellor is there as a resource to help the client become their own counsellor, so that the client progresses towards being able to offer themselves honesty, empathy, and compassion. The counsellor offers their honest, empathic, compassionate presence to the client not to re-parent or create a cosy dependency, but rather to enable the client to do likewise for self. Thus, the counsellor might say at session 1: 'Well, we've got X sessions. I know that might seem like a lot, but it's amazing how fast it can go, so where would you like to start?'

It is particularly important to remind the client when four or fewer sessions remain. For example, you might say, 'I'm aware that we have four sessions after today. How does that sit with you? Is there anything in particular that you want to get to before we end?' This initiates the ending phase and work of counselling. It also often mobilizes clients to stop putting off work on issues that they may have been avoiding. In addition, it is a good idea to listen for and explore termination feelings that the client raises, regardless of when these come up in counselling, and to suggest to the client that it would be useful to reserve enough time at the end to properly explore their experience of ending.

Having done this, it can be useful for the counsellor to reserve some time on their own or in supervision to reflect on how they and the client are likely to experience the ending of this counselling. For example, given the client's history, presenting issues, and progress towards resolving those issues, how are they likely to experience ending? What kinds are difficulties might they experience with ending? Are they likely to feel abandoned? And what about me (the counsellor)? What issues do I have with endings in my life in general? How have I been touched or changed by this client? What will I be able to say in the last session to this client that is both authentic and likely to be helpful to them?

3. Exploring the experience of ending. Clients vary widely in the meaning they attach to ending counselling. Some clients are apprehensive, fearful of 'back-sliding' after finishing. Other clients have a sense of readiness and excitement about the prospect of facing challenges on their own. Feelings of emptiness or loss are common and sometimes quite poignant (Barge & Elliott, 2016). If the termination is externally imposed, some clients will feel unready and may experience the ending as abandonment or rejection, in which case some effort may be needed to extend counselling or to find alternative care. Because of these widely varying reactions, it's best to make no assumptions about how a client feels about ending, and to find an appropriate moment at least once during this set of final sessions to simply ask them, 'I'm wondering what comes up inside for you when you think about ending?'

4. Looking ahead. From the beginning, the counsellor has been thinking about the client as an active participant in counselling, who is soon going to have to manage on their own. Therefore, in the final one or two sessions, regardless of whether the client feels entirely ready or not, it's usually a good idea to offer the client an opportunity to explore their continuing and future life projects: 'What's your sense right now of what is next for you? Is there anything left unfinished here? What are you planning to continue working on?' To the extent that such continuing issues are an important part of the client's experience of ending, they are explored, perhaps harking back to the original shared understanding of the interrupted life projects that led the client to seek counselling in the first place.

5. Doing the ending: Final session subtasks. When the final session arrives, it's often useful to help the client review the ending work from the previous sessions. In addition, there are three ending subtasks that may be very useful for clients. First, the counsellor can help the client *explore their sense of progress* (or lack of it) over the course of their counselling. This often involves a particular type of empathic exploration in which the client compares their current and previous psychological states. Thus, the counsellor might say, 'I wonder, now, as you look back to when you were starting counselling, what feels different to you now, as opposed to when you started?' Often, clients do not fully realize how depressed or stuck they were until they are no longer depressed or stuck. At the same time, the counsellor can help the client develop a fuller understanding of their current state by comparing it to how they were before counselling, moving back and forth between current and previous states, so that each sheds light on the other. This provides a fuller understanding and appreciation of *both* states than would have been possible if the exploration were limited to one or the other. In the process, the counsellor helps the client to reflect on how they got from point A to point B and to consolidate a coherent, emotionally-grounded story about this process.

A second potentially useful final session subtask is *normalizing post-ending distress*. Barge and Elliott (2016) state that clients often reported that after the last session of counselling they were surprised by unexpected difficult feelings, especially of sadness or anxiety. Therefore, we suggest that it might be beneficial to let clients know about this possibility, and to normalize the experience by letting them know that this is quite common and natural.

The third useful final session subtask is a *mutual sharing* of the experience of counselling and ending. The counsellor starts by asking, with genuine curiosity, 'Now, as we come to an end, how do you feel about the work you've done here, and also about us ending today?' But, then, after hearing the client out and carefully reflecting their experiences, it's generally completely appropriate and helpful for the EFC counsellor to disclose their experience of ending, as well as some positive experience of working with the client. For example, they might say, 'You know, if I take a moment to check inside with myself, I find myself feeling both a bit sad for us to end, but at the same time also excited for you going forward. I know it has been hard work for you and sometimes painful, and I feel privileged to have been able to help you in working through all that.' In general, this is likely to require some personal work by the counsellor in order to clarify their experience of the ending and the client's current state. It is vital, whatever the counsellor chooses to disclose to the client, that it be both genuine *and* truly facilitative to the client. For example, it is important to display genuine pleasure with the client's progress, but that doesn't mean you should make something up that you don't believe!

6. Post-ending reflection. In a study of clients' experiences of ending EFC, Barge and Elliott (2016) found that the ending process extended past the last session of counselling, as clients continued to reflect on their counselling and make sense out of it. Of course, counsellors don't hear about this, unless clients let them know later, either through spontaneous letters or emails, or through later returning to counselling. For this reason, in some settings it can be a good idea to routinely follow up with clients by collecting quantitative or qualitative outcome data.

A final point is recognizing that counselling changes both the client and the counsellor, especially if it is successful. For this reason, it's a good idea to use your personal supervision or reflective journal to create a meaning perspective on the work you've done with each client: What am I left with after finishing with this client? Is there anything left unfinished? What have I learned here? What went well? What would I do differently with similar clients or issues in the future? For the counsellor, every client that you truly come to know adds not only to your level of experience, empathy, skill, and confidence, but more importantly to the sum total of your human experience; it enlarges you as a human being. This is true whether you have been practising counselling for six months or 40 years, but it is perhaps most poignant when ending with your first client in EFC.

Variations in Ending

Clearly, the ideal situation involves a client having successfully resolved their main presenting difficulties within initially agreed-upon time limits. However, life is often not so simple. Here are some common alternative endings, together with suggestions for facilitating each.

1. Finishing early. To begin with, even if client and counsellor have agreed to a certain number of sessions, the client may complete their work before that number of sessions is reached, as Bethany did. Clients often complete their projected therapeutic work more quickly than expected, to the surprise and sometimes dismay of their counsellors. If the client feels ready to end sooner than originally agreed to, it is generally a good idea to support this. After all, the client is the active agent in their counselling. Like other humanistic approaches to counselling, EFC does not subscribe to the psychodynamic concept of 'flight into health' (Frick, 1999). In other words, from an EFC point of view, sudden, unexpected improvements in general do not mean that clients are trying to leave counselling in order to avoid having to deal with their difficult experiences.

Nevertheless, the counsellor will in any case be curious about and want to explore the client's sense of progress and readiness. If the counsellor harbours doubts about the client's motives or readiness for ending, a useful possibility is to offer to spread out the last session or two or to offer a one-month follow-up session, to make sure that the client is really ready to end. If the client is being overly optimistic, this will give them enough time for problems to crop up, and also allow the client to continue without losing face. In general, clients are encouraged to explore their experience of improvement and, if necessary, to make explicit choices about whether or not they want to continue counselling. EFC counsellors recognize and accept the fact that this may not be the right time to work on particularly difficult issues, and will validate their clients' decisions, while still leaving the door open should the client decide they want to come back.

2. Running out of sessions before being done. Because we live in an era in which mental health services are under-funded, we have to live increasingly with the rationing of counselling in the form of rather severe time limits, often as few as six sessions. Such externally imposed time limits mean that many clients will still be clinically distressed when they run out of sessions. Sometimes it is possible to extend the counselling, but if not, it may be necessary to refer them elsewhere. This is a difficult situation, and such limits need to be discussed from the beginning. Doing so makes it possible for client and counsellor to focus on less painful, more circumscribed problems that can be addressed within the time limits, if that is the client's preference. We have found that clients receiving EFC in such situations sometimes break up their counselling into multiple brief episodes of discrete pieces of therapeutic work, returning after the required interval to pick up where they left off.

3. Running out of things to work on but not feeling ready to end. Some clients reach the point of having improved substantially and having little to work on in therapy, but may still not feel ready to end. These clients may fear relapse or may lack a network of supportive others, or they may simply find it beneficial to have someone to check in with periodically. For these clients, a useful strategy is to suggest meeting less frequently: every other week, monthly, or when the client feels they need to. It is perfectly OK for a client to continue intermittently in counselling for several years, with EFC providing an occasional check-up function.

4. Giving up on therapy. Another possibility is that the client may wish to stop counselling because they no longer see it as useful, either because they feel it is the wrong kind of counselling for them or because they come to see their problems as too intractable, painful or difficult to work on productively. Such decisions, however painful, need to be explored wherever possible, but should be understood and respected. In these cases, the therapist needs to develop and communicate an empathic understanding of why it feels important not to go on. For example, one depressed client had resolved most of her difficulties and stopped therapy because she feared stirring up problems in her marital relationship. Although she was not entirely satisfied with this relationship, it was still better than her previous marriage to an emotionally and physically abusive man. Understanding her situation allowed the counsellor to appreciate and validate this as a reasonable decision on the part of the client.

5. Open-door ending. Finally, and especially in private practice settings, the counsellor can offer future sessions if and when the client needs it, encouraging the client to come into and out of counselling as they need it over a period of time (Cummings & Sayama, 1995). This gives clients a sense of control over their counselling and is particularly appropriate for clients with difficult, long-standing issues.

Jonah Finishes Counselling

Jonah arrives late for his last session and comments that he is at a whole new level of awareness, feels he is moving in the right direction, not reacting as fast as he used to, and thinking before he reacts. He says that he has changed and is now separating his self-worth from the amount of love and recognition he perceives he is getting from others. He recognizes that people biting his head off for no reason may not have anything to do with him and that there is no need to panic. He is more secure now, not so shaky, and feels relieved that he is able to be more disengaged when people get angry around him. His depression has lifted and he is feeling more hopeful. He attributes the change to counselling and being able to deal with his feelings towards his mother.

By the end of counselling, Jonah has tentatively changed his view of his critical mother from someone who deliberately hurt him to someone who might not have been aware of hurting him: 'Perhaps she was not aware that she was hurting me.'

In addition, he has begun to tolerate his anger towards her and has allowed his sadness. The main goal of counselling, agreed upon at the beginning, has been to overcome his depression by dealing with his mother's effect on his self-worth. By grieving not having had the mother he would have liked to have had, he has been able to let go of a lot of bad feelings he has carried for years. His view of himself has become that of someone whose scars are healing; he no longer believes he is a bad person. In the last session, after reviewing what had happened during counselling and how much Jonah had changed, Jonah thanks the therapist, who says she will miss working with him. They laugh about how he is so much better now, indicated by the fact he can cry. They end by wishing each other well and the therapist says he shouldn't hesitate to call in future if he wants any booster sessions.

Further Exploration

Reading

Barge, A., & Elliott, R. (2016). Clients' experiences of ending person-centred/experiential time limited therapy. Unpublished manuscript, Counselling Unit, University of Strathclyde, Glasgow, Scotland. Available at: www.dropbox.com/s/ghddw0ksv3g6fjl/_Barge%20%26%20Elliott%20Endings%202016.docx?dl=0

Frick, W. B. (1999). Flight into health: A new interpretation. *Journal of Humanistic Psychology, 39*, 58–81.

Greenberg, L. S. (2002). Termination of experiential therapy. *Journal of Psychotherapy Integration, 12*(3), 358–363.

Watching

Greenberg, L.S. (2007). *Emotion-Focused Therapy over Time*. American Psychological Association Videos. [See session 6 for an example of the final session of short-term EFC]

Reflecting

1. Spend some time reflecting on your experience of endings in your life. Can you think of some that were more difficult than others? Try writing a bit about what made them difficult. Now see if you can think of one or two 'good' endings you've experienced. What made them good or satisfying? What attitudes towards ending in general do you think you've taken away from these experiences? How might this affect your practice as a counsellor?

2. What kinds of difficulties might you have in ending with a client who doesn't feel ready to end? What about a client who simply 'disappears off the face of the earth' (i.e., stops coming to sessions and doesn't answer your messages)?

10

Next Steps in Emotion-Focused Counselling

Chapter Outline

Overview of Chapter

Other Aspects of Emotion-Focused Counselling

Adaptations for Different Client Populations

A Brief User-friendly Summary of Process Research on EFC

Methods for Monitoring Your EFC Practice

Recommendations for Further Learning and Practice

Conclusion

Overview of Chapter

The aim of this chapter is to provide a bridge for those who want to go on to develop their practice as emotion-focused counsellors. Thus, we offer brief overviews of material not covered in previous chapters, including other tasks, adaptations for different client populations, research on change processes in EFC, methods of outcome and process monitoring, and suggestions for further learning and practice.

Other Aspects of Emotion-Focused Counselling

Other EFC tasks. In this brief overview of EFC theory and practice, we have had by necessity to focus on a set of key tasks organized by phase of counselling. On the one hand, we have briefly presented *experiential tasks* like Narrative Retelling in Chapter 4, Evocative Unfolding and Focusing in Chapter 5, and Empathic Affirmation in Chapter 8. These tasks come out of the Person-Centred-Experiential counselling tradition and are also important in EFC. On the other hand, we went into some depth on different forms of chair work, including Two Chair Work for conflict splits (Chapter 6), and Empty Chair Work for unresolved relational issues (Chapter 7) and Compassionate Self-Soothing (Chapter 8). These tasks have been adapted from the Gestalt therapy and Psychodrama traditions. These two sets of tasks are the primary ones used in EFC and provide a good starter set for learning EFC.

However, we have given short shrift to four more specialized tasks that have been developed or assimilated by EFC practitioners and researchers and are worth a look. These were listed in Table 5.1; most are described in more detail elsewhere (e.g., Elliott et al., 2004).

First, *Relational Dialogue* is used to repair alliance difficulties or ruptures (Elliott & MacDonald, 2020; Elliott et al., 2004). We distinguish between two types of relational difficulties: *confrontation difficulties*, in which the client makes a direct or implicit complaint or expresses dissatisfaction with the counsellor, the counselling itself or some aspect of it, and *withdrawal difficulties*, in which the client disengages from the work of therapy (for example, by coming late to sessions or avoiding therapeutic work; Safran & Muran, 2000). When this happens, the counsellor always assumes that they have in some way contributed to the difficulty, and engages with the client in an open discussion of the part each has played in the difficulty.

Second, *Clearing a Space* is a task closely related to Focusing and is used when the client is unable to find a productive focus of attention for the session. This can involve either feeling overwhelmed by numerous concerns, or, conversely, being unable to identify what to work on in the session (Elliott et al., 2004; Grindler Katonah, 1999). In Clearing a Space, the counsellor guides the client through a kind of Focusing process in which they identify their various concerns and imagine setting them aside one at a time, either in the counselling room or in an imaginary safe space. (We offered a brief version of this as an exercise at the end of Chapter 5.)

Third, *Meaning Re-Creation* was developed by Clarke (1989, 1991) for use with clients who are in an overwhelmed, angry state of protest because of unexpected traumatic events, such as tragic losses or betrayals. This *meaning protest* marker (Elliott et al., 2004) is somewhat similar to the unresolved relationship issues marker for Empty Chair Work; however, in this case the client's emotions are not blocked but are instead strongly aroused to the point of emotion dysregulation, making Empty Chair Work inappropriate, at least at that moment. In this task, the counsellor helps the client to symbolize the traumatic experience and the *cherished belief* that has been violated by the trauma. Meaning Re-Creation work helps clients use language and metaphor to regulate their overwhelming emotions during a crisis, paving the way for later Empty Chair Work (Clarke, 1993). (For more, see Elliott et al., 2004.)

Finally, although developed by Gary Prouty (1998), a student of Carl Rogers and a person-centred counsellor, *Contact Work* also fits neatly into the framework of EFC tasks. The marker, *loss of psychological contact*, occurs when the client is having a psychotic, dissociative or panic episode in the session. The counsellor offers the client concrete, specific process reflections (referred to as *contact reflections*) of what the client is doing ('You look away', 'George is rocking back and forth') or of the immediate situation ('The carpet is blue', 'A car is driving by outside'). These responses gradually bring the client back into psychological contact through a series of stages. Adding this task to EFC means that it can be used with clients with psychotic or dissociative processes. (For more, see Sanders, 2007.)

Other modalities of EFC. In this book, we have focused on EFC for individuals, as opposed to couples and families. However, *emotion-focused therapy for couples* (EFT-C) is a well-established approach that helps members of a couple access and express under-lying attachment-oriented emotions, such as sadness and separation anxiety (Greenberg & Goldman, 2008; Greenberg & Johnson, 1988; Johnson, 2004). With an extensive research literature, this approach has been found to be effective in increasing marital satisfaction (e.g., Johnson & Greenberg, 1985; Johnson et al., 1999) and other presenting difficulties, including depression. Today, EFT-C is recognized as one of the most effec-tive approaches in resolving relationship distress (Baucom, Shoham, Mueser, Daiuto, & Stickle, 1998; Johnson et al., 1999). Furthermore, a set of couples counselling markers have been identified and studied: attachment injuries, identity injuries, and dominance inter-actions have been defined and studied (Greenberg & Goldman, 2008), while attachment injury/forgiveness work has been investigated and modelled (Greenberg & Woldarsky Meneses, 2019).

A more recent development is *Emotion-Focused Family Therapy* (EFFT), which primarily takes the form of parent training interventions where the parent is helped to learn how to become more facilitative in their interactions with their troubled children, typically through helping them overcome blocks to their empathy (LaFrance, Henderson, & Mayman, 2019). There is an emerging body of evidence to support this offshoot of EFC (e.g., Foroughe et al., 2019), as well as a closely related approach, attachment-based family therapy (Diamond, Diamond, & Levy, 2014).

Adaptations for Different Client Populations

EFC is *transdiagnostic*, which means that we understand that it works across a wide range of client populations or presenting problems, including depression, anxiety, eating difficulties, and so on (Timulak et al., 2020). However, we also assume that different client populations will present with somewhat different task markers, and that a particular EFC task may have a somewhat different focus for, say, depression as opposed to social anxiety. Thus, when EFC counsellors approach a new client population, they assume that the approach will need to be adapted, both in general and for specific clients.

Depression. For example, EFC was originally developed for work with depressed clients, where depressed states are understood as a form of stuck or blocked pro-cess involving a weak/bad self-experiencer who collapses in the face of an angry or contemptuous inner critic. For clients with this presentation, it's generally a good idea to start by providing clients with strong empathy, which helps them explore the sources of their depression. Focusing (see Chapter 4) is often useful for helping clients begin to access blocked emotions or ground overly conceptual processing in the body. However, the most important tasks for depressed clients are Two Chair Work for harsh self-critical conflict splits (see Chapter 6) and Empty Chair Work for unresolved relationship issues (see Chapter 7). (For more, see Greenberg & Watson, 2005; Salgado, Cunha, & Monteiro, 2019; Watson, Goldman, & Greenberg, 2007.)

Complex trauma/interpersonal injury. Another early application of EFC was with complex trauma, which occurs in clients who have survived extended histories of interpersonal abuse. Jonah, presented as one of our two running examples throughout this book, is an example of a client with a complex trauma presentation. Clients like Jonah often experience a range of interpersonal and self-related difficulties, including emotion over- and under-regulation, and chronic anger towards self and others. For such clients, alliance formation and relational dialogue are critical for helping repair deep-seated emotion schemes of others as malevolent or at best unhelpful. In addition, self-interruption splits (see Chapter 6) are common and must be dealt with before proceeding to work on the trauma itself, via Narrative Retelling (see Chapter 4) and Empty Chair Work (Chapter 7). Meaning creation and space clearing (both discussed earlier in this chapter) can also be useful at times. (For more, see Paivio & Pascual-Leone, 2010.)

Anxiety. Somewhat different versions of EFC have recently been developed for generalized anxiety (involving excessive worry) and social anxiety (involving excessive fear of other people). Bethany, our other running example, came to counselling to work on her social anxiety, or fear of other people. Anxiety difficulties tend to revolve around stuck emotions of shame, guilt, and vulnerability. Clients present with *anxiety splits,* in which a critical/coercive part of the self, variously referred to as a *worrier* (Timulak & McElvaney, 2017) or a *coach-critic-guard* (Elliott & Shahar, 2019), regularly warns the experiencer of dangers, causing them to feel anxious or afraid. However, this is only the surface layer of the client's process; underneath, there is a harsh, critical conflict that continually reinforces underlying guilt or shame, and also unresolved traumatic experiences, such as chronic humiliation or loss/abandonment. For this reason, Empty Chair Work and Compassionate Self-Soothing are both important tasks for this client population. (For more, see Elliott & Shahar, 2019; Timulak & McElvaney, 2017; Watson & Greenberg, 2017.)

In addition to these three common presentations, versions of EFC have also been developed for eating difficulties (Dolhanty & LaFrance, 2019) and high-functioning autism (Robinson & Elliott, 2017). Beyond this, a group format of EFC has recently emerged, focusing on self-criticism (Thompson & Girz, 2020).

Transdiagnostic EFC. However, we don't want to give you the wrong impression. Just because we are talking about different client presentations doesn't mean that EFC counsellors are heavily into psychiatric diagnosis and the medical model. We are not interested in psychiatric labels or medicalizing distress, but we are interested in clients' emotional experiences, like being depressed or weighed down, or tormented by worries about bad things that could happen. Overall, though, we see that the many different client populations bring common emotional difficulties, such as secondary emotion responses covering up adaptive responses, maladaptive emotion schemes, undifferentiated or undersymbolized emotions, and difficulties with affect regulation (both under- and over-). Furthermore, clients need to be treated as whole persons, each with their own idiosyncratic histories and unique combinations of emotion difficulties. In other words, the person is not the symptom, and diagnostic categories can do more harm than good in counselling, especially if we take them too seriously. Ultimately, we see EFC as *transdiagnostic* (to use a currently trendy jargon term; see Greenberg, in press; Timulak et al., 2020), because in the end the basic in-session processes and tasks are the same regardless of diagnosis. All use empathy, focusing, narrative work, various kinds of chair work, case formulation, and so on.

On the other hand, we do find that people with common presenting issues, such as anxiety or eating difficulties, do have certain common characteristics so that grouping them into diagnostic categories does help to some degree, as long as we don't treat diagnostic categories as more than rough approximations that can provide broad understandings that need to be filled in with the richness that each client presents. A good starting place and practice is to replace the word 'disorder' with 'difficulties' wherever possible (for example, anxiety difficulties). Clients come to counselling not because of their disorders but because something is difficult in their lives.

Preventive approaches. One of the most pressing needs within the larger emotion-focused approach is the development of programmes of skills training in emotional literacy and experientially-based psycho-education programmes on how to utilize, manage, and change emotion (Greenberg, 2015). Probably a key time to introduce such training, especially in managing and transforming emotion, is in adolescence, when emotions often become problematic. Emotion awareness is the basic skill that needs to be started in the home and with young children, ideally followed by more extensive work on emotion regulation and transformation from adolescence onwards. In order to help develop emotional competence in children, it's important for adults, parents, and teachers to be aware and accepting of their own emotions, the first requirement for an effective *emotion coach*. For this, training of adolescents and young adults may be the best entry point, so that as they mature and become parents and teachers, they will become good emotion coaches for the next generation.

Thus, preventive or emotion coaching skill development programmes are appropriate for children, adolescents, young adults, and parents. Regardless of level, such programmes can focus on learning about and practising attending to one's emotions; this will help the person to become more compassionate to self and others, to learn to let go of resentments, to regulate emotion, to reflect on emotions, and to change emotions that are problematic. All of these are crucial steps in becoming an EFC counsellor and in applying EFC work more broadly. Our hope is to help promote these sorts of developments.

A Brief User-friendly Summary of Process Research on EFC

As we noted in Chapter 1, there now is solid evidence for the efficacy and effectiveness of EFT for individuals who are depressed or anxious, who have eating difficulties, or who have experienced interpersonal injury or complex trauma. In addition, there is a substantial amount of research on the process of change in EFC, validating the key idea that reflection on aroused emotion, and the expression of core pain is beneficial and leads to positive outcomes in counselling. (See reviews by Elliott et al., 2013; Elliott et al., in press; Greenberg, in press; Timulak et al., 2019.)

In terms of process research, what appears critical is emotional expression in conjunction with self-reflective processing. In other words, both the 'heart' and the 'head' are essential for change. Further, it is the *quantity* and *productivity* of emotional arousal that is important and not just emotional arousal alone. In addition, EFC proposes that the best way to change an emotion (for example, maladaptive shame) is with another emotion (for example, assertive anger). Extensive quantitative research on the role of emotion in therapeutic change has consistently demonstrated a relationship between in-session emotional activation and client outcome. A recent systematic review of process-outcome studies by Pascual-Leone and Yeryomenko (2017) showed a robust relationship between in-session emotional experiencing, as measured by the Experiencing Scale (EXP) (Klein, Mathieu-Coughlan & Kiesler, 1986), and therapeutic gain in a range of forms of counselling, including psychodynamic, cognitive, and experiential. These findings suggest that processing one's bodily feelings and deepening these in counselling may well be a core ingredient of change, regardless of approach.

More specifically in EFC, process-outcome research on EFC for depression has consistently supported the value of paying attention to and making sense of emotion. Studies have shown that higher emotional arousal in the middle of counselling, together with self-reflection on the aroused emotion and deeper emotional processing late in counselling, predict good outcomes (Pos, Greenberg, & Warwar, 2009). For example, high emotional arousal plus high reflection on aroused emotion distinguished good from poor outcome cases, pointing to the importance of combining arousal and meaning construction (Missirlian et al., 2005). Emotion-focused counselling thus appears to work by enhancing the type of emotional processing that involves helping people to experience and accept their emotions, and then make sense of them.

Beyond this, however, EFC process-outcome research has also found that approach, arousal, acceptance, and tolerance of emotional experience is necessary but not sufficient for change; there must also be emotion transformation, that is, changing emotion with emotion by accessing core pain, as we described in Chapter 3 and illustrated in Chapters 6, 7 and 8. Optimum emotional processing involves in addition the integration of thought (cognition) and feeling (emotion) into a meaning perspective or new narrative (Greenberg, 2015; Greenberg & Pascual-Leone, 1995). Once contact with emotional experience is achieved, clients must also treat that experience as information, accessing and exploring it, reflecting on it, and finding words for it. In the end, it's important for them to use their emotions to make sense of themselves and their situations, while also accessing their other internal emotional resources, such as assertive anger and self-compassion, in order to help transform their stuck, maladaptive emotion responses.

Methods for Monitoring Your EFC Practice

You've probably already gathered that research has always been an important aspect of EFC. Beyond this, we recommend that EFC counsellors integrate appropriate research methods into their practice. Ideally, these will help you reflect on your skill level and support you in developing further in the practice of EFC. You can also use outcome measures to see if your clients are changing over the course of counselling. In this section we'll present some simple, free (!) methods that can be useful for this. Some of these are included as appendices in this book; other useful counselling monitoring and research tools can be accessed at the websites links provided below.

EFT Therapist Session Form (ETSF, v6.0; Elliott, 2019) (see Appendix 1). This is a useful form for recording your process notes and for rating your sessions from the point of view of the concepts introduced in this book, including EFC principles (see Chapter 1), client emotion processing modes (Chapter 2), and counselling tasks (Chapters 4 and 5). As such, it provides an opportunity for self-supervision, an aid to formal supervision, and a record (both qualitative and quantitative) of what happened in the session.

Person-Centred and Experiential Psychotherapy Scale – EFT Supplement, Therapist Version (PCEPS-EFT-T, v1.0) (see Appendix 2). The original version of the PCEPS (Freire, Elliott, & Westwell, 2014) assessed person-centred-experiential counselling skills and was adopted as the competence measure for Person-Centred-Experiential Counselling for Depression training in England and Wales. Unfortunately, this measure was not specific enough to be useful for evaluating counsellor competence in EFC; therefore, an EFC-supplement instrument (the PCEPS-EFT-5) was developed, to support EFC research and to help evaluate counsellors and psychotherapists who have submitted recordings to be evaluated for counsellor accreditation following requirements set by the International Society for Emotion-Focused Therapy (ISEFT). The PCEPS-EFT-T is a counsellor self-report version of this instrument that you can use to evaluate your EFC practice on five dimensions: *empathic attunement, marker identification, emotion deepening, appropriate use of EFT tasks*, and *EFT case formulation*. Each dimension is rated on a detailed six-point rating scale, ranging from 1 ('Much improvement needed: Beginner, doesn't have concept yet') to 6 ('Excellent implementation: Trainer level of skill: Consistent and creative'). Accreditation requires performance at level 4 ('Adequate implementation: Does reasonably well, although there is still room for improvement') on all five dimensions.

Outcome Measures. It's a good idea to use a standardized general outcome measure, before therapy and every eight or 10 sessions. We like the *CORE Outcome Measure*

(Barkham et al., 2001; available at: www.core-systems.co.uk/home.html) because it's free, well-researched, and measures emotional distress in a general sort of way. Another possibility is to use a brief individualized problem measure, filled out by the client before each session. Such measures ask clients to identify the major problem areas that they want to change, and to rate how much these problems have bothered them over the past week; one example is the *Personal Questionnaire* (Elliott et al., 2016). These measures are more work to create than standardized general measures, but they are more in keeping with EFC and other humanistic approaches because they do not force the client to use pre-determined items. Also, they are short enough that they can be filled out before each session, so that they can be used to track client progress over the course of counselling. (For more on the Personal Questionnaire, see: http://experiential-researchers.org/instruments/elliott/pqprocedure.html.)

Counselling process instruments. It can also be useful to ask clients about important things happening in their counselling. For example, the *Helpful Aspects of Therapy (HAT) Form* (Llewelyn, 1988) (see Appendix 3) is a qualitative, open-ended questionnaire that asks the client to describe the most helpful or important thing that happened in a counselling session. To this can be added a measure of the working alliance between client and counsellor, which can be administered after every session, or every three to five sessions; the revised 12-item short form of the Working Alliance Inventory (WAI-12-R; Hatcher & Gillaspy, 2006) is the most frequently used counselling relationship measure and highly consistent with EFC (it was developed by Horvath & Greenberg, 1989). (The WAI-12-R can be obtained at: https://wai.profhorvath.com/downloads; the recommended versions are: SF Hatcher Client and SF Hatcher Therapist.)

Recordings. Finally, audio- or video-recordings are essential for learning EFC. In addition to being required for EFC supervision, they also allow you to look at your practice more closely and to learn from your clients' immediate responses to what you offer them in sessions.

Recommendations for Further Learning and Practice

Learning resources. Having reached the end of this book, what further reading and other resources do we recommend? That depends on what you want. Table 10.1 presents an annotated list of books, videos and websites that will help you learn more about EFC. Part A lists books, which range from very simple (Timulak, 2015) to fairly technical (Greenberg & Goldman, 2018). However, in EFC we don't want you to take our word for it; we feel that it is important to actually look at the practice, so in Part B of Table 10.1 we provide a starter list of EFC videos and encourage you to see the practice for yourself. The first three listed (Elliott, 2016; Greenberg , 2020a, 2020b) are relatively inexpensive; however, the other two are expensive. You may need to borrow one or get your university or training institute to purchase them or to subscribe to a video streaming service. Finally, in Part C of Table 10.1 we've listed a couple of websites where you can find more information about EFC. (Don't be put off by the fact that these resources all refer to Emotion–Focused *Therapy*; there is no difference between what we have referred to here as *EFC* and what is elsewhere called *EFT*. A word of warning, however: there is *no* connection between EFC and the 'other' EFT, referred to as the Emotional Freedom Technique.)

TABLE 10.1 *Annotated list of resources for learning more about EFC*

Resource	Description
A. Key Books	
Timulak (2015). *Transforming emotional pain in psychotherapy* (Routledge)	Straightforward simplified presentation focusing on emotional deepening model.
Elliott, Watson, Goldman & Greenberg (2004). *Learning emotion-focused therapy* (APA)	Clear but detailed, encyclopaedic coverage of EFC tasks, focused on learning process.
Goldman & Greenberg (2014). *Case formulation in emotion-focused therapy* (APA)	Complex model of EFC case formulation; systematic presentation of most recent EFC theory.
Paivio & Pascual-Leone (2010). *Emotion-focused therapy for complex trauma* (APA)	A must if you work with a client population with complex trauma.
Greenberg & Goldman (2018). *Clinical handbook of emotion-focused therapy* (APA)	Fairly technical but the most up-to-date source on the broad range of EFC theory and practice.
Watson, Goldman & Greenberg (2007). *Case studies in emotion-focused therapy for depression* (APA)	Contains extensive transcripts of EFC sessions that you can read aloud for deliberate practice to build your skills.
B. Recommended Videos	
Elliott (2016). *Understanding emotion-focused therapy* (Counselling Channel)	Video of narrative retelling, empty chair work and compassionate self-soothing with a male client.
Greenberg (2020a). *EFT: Working with core emotion* (Counselling Channel)	Video of two chair work and empathic affirmation of core pain with a female client.
Greenberg (2020b). *EFT: Working with current and historical trauma* (Counselling Channel)	Video of empty chair work for complex relational trauma with a female client.
Greenberg (2007). *Emotion-focused therapy over time* (APA)	Expensive but essential for mastering EFC; includes version with therapist commentary.
Paivio (2013). *Emotion-focused therapy for complex trauma* (APA)	A master trauma counsellor in an initial EFC session with a client with complex trauma (expensive).
C. Websites	
International Society for Emotion-Focused Therapy (ISEFT): www.iseft.org/	Contains a range of information about EFC/EFT, including lists of trainings, therapists, and so on.

Training. The resources listed in Table 10.1 will take you further, but to really learn EFC you will need to do systematic training. Sometimes, you can find this training (or parts of it) within a counselling or psychotherapy training course. In general, however, you will need to sign up for workshop-based training, usually at the post-qualification or continuing professional development level. Elliott et al. (2004) described a multifaceted training programme to help counsellors learn EFC, consisting of the following:

- Self-selection for basic experiential capacities and interests;
- Safe, supportive but stimulating training context;
- Didactic learning about EFC theory and practice, including lectures and readings;
- Observation of live and recorded examples;
- Supervised practice in the counsellor role, with both technique and personal development;
- Direct experience in the client role, in order to experience the effects of task interventions from the inside; and
- Reflexivity, supported by self-observation/evaluation, client feedback, and participation in continuing learning and skill development.

Because of the critical role of empathy, counsellors learning EFC will either have previously learned person-centred counselling or will need to focus on the person-centred relational attitudes and skills of accurate empathy, unconditional positive regard, and genuineness/transparency early in their EFC training. EFC training typically begins with emotion theory (see Chapters 2 and 3 of this book), ideally with experiential exercises to help participants recognize different emotion processes in themselves. When it comes to the tasks, training sometimes begins with the less process-guiding tasks of empathic exploration - Narrative Retelling, Focusing and Evocative Unfolding - before shifting to the different forms of chair work. Training in each task typically begins with didactic instruction and group discussion about the task, in particular its markers. This is followed by perceptual training, that is, looking at videos showing how counsellors pick up and facilitate the task, along with skill practice in both client and counsellor roles. After this, trainees are closely supervised with actual clients, which we discuss below.

EFC supervision. Consistent with its origins in counselling process research, and in contrast to typical modes of supervision in person-centred counselling today, EFC supervision is primarily focused on careful review of recordings of counselling sessions, ideally video-recordings (Greenberg & Tomescu, 2017). Together, supervisee and supervisor review the recording of part of a session selected by the supervisee to illustrate a question or concern they have brought. For example, in our experience, one of the most common supervision questions is 'What more could I have done here to help my client deepen their emotions?' At other times, supervisees bring questions about a specific task ('How could I have done better here with empty chair work?') or case formulation ('I'm confused: What is going on with this client?'). Together, supervisor and supervisee listen carefully for (a) important elements of what the client presents (markers and micro-markers); (b) the wording and manner in which the counsellor delivers their responses; and (c) how the client immediately reacts to the counsellor's responses.

From this, it can be seen that much of the focus is on helping counsellors to develop their perceptual skills for identifying important aspects of the counselling process. Other modes of EFC supervision include:

- Case formulation of how the client's difficult process works;
- Having the supervisee embody (role play) their client while the supervisor takes the role of counsellor;
- As appropriate, personal work on stuck places or blocks that are interfering in the counsellor's work with clients; this may involve self-critical or self-interruption splits, or unfinished business with the client; and
- Recommended readings to support the counsellor's learning.

For more on EFC supervision, see Greenberg and Tomescu (2017).

Accreditation. Standards and procedures for becoming certified in EFC/EFT have been developed by the International Society for Emotion-Focused Therapy (see: www.iseft.org/page-18205). In order to be certified in EFC, counsellors must complete between eight and 13 days (depending on the region in which they practise) of official EFC workshop training. In addition, they must receive at least 16 hours supervision in EFT from an accredited EFT supervisor. Finally, they must submit two recordings to their supervisor for formal evaluation. (The recordings must include chair work with two different clients, be accompanied by a written case formulation, and be passed by the supervisor.)

Conclusion

So there you have it. We've presented a brief introduction to Emotion-Focused Counselling, in which we've tried to make EFC theory and practice as clear as possible, while also grounding it in real-world practice. We realize that we've covered a lot of material, impossible to assimilate all at once, so we want you to be patient with yourself. Learning any approach to counselling is challenging and can be intimidating; it takes time, and you may feel overwhelmed or deskilled at times. That's perfectly natural. *Learning* EFC takes time, personal development, and lots of practice and supervision. *Mastering* EFC can take many years, but you've got to start somewhere, and there will be many adventures along the way.

It has been our pleasure here to provide you with a flavour of the general parameters, theory, and various phases of the practice of Emotion-Focused Counselling, illustrated by its application with two different clients. While we recognize that EFC is not for everyone, either as counsellor or client, we sincerely hope that your EFC journey will not stop here, and that we have whetted your appetite for more, or at least helped you decide whether you want to go further. This is because we have personally experienced the transforming power of emotion in our own lives, as we encountered our own personal stucknesses and emotional pain, allowed ourselves to stay with the pain and to find what hurt the most, which then helped us move forward out of the stuckness into new more adaptive emotions. It's also because EFC has transformed our way of working with clients, allowing us to feel truly grounded as counsellors and authentically connected to ourselves and our clients. Being able to work in this way and to offer training in it to others has provided us with immense satisfaction and personal meaning. We hope that in this book we've communicated at least some of the power and excitement of EFC.

Appendix 1

EFT Therapist Session Form (v6.0) (11/19, ©R. Elliott)

CASE_____   SESSION_____   LENGTH_____DATE_____
THERAPIST_____

Outcome Measure:_____ Score:_____ Signal Status: W G Y R

I. Process Notes

1. Brief summary of main episodes and events of session:

2. Unusual Within-therapy Events (e.g., late, interruptions, challenges, out-of-mode):

3. Important Extra-therapy Events (e.g., relationships, work, injury/illness, changes in medication, self-help efforts):

4. Ideas for next time (from self & supervision):

II. Overall Session Ratings

1. Please rate how helpful or hindering to your client you think this session was overall. (Check one answer only) THIS SESSION WAS:	____ 1. Extremely hindering ____ 2. Greatly hindering ____ 3. Moderately hindering ____ 4. Slightly hindering ____ 5. Neither helpful nor hindering; neutral ____ 6. Slightly helpful ____ 7. Moderately helpful ____ 8. Greatly helpful ____ 9. Extremely helpful
2. How do you feel about the session you have just completed with your client?	____ 1. Perfect ____ 2. Excellent ____ 3. Very good ____ 4. Pretty good ____ 5. Fair ____ 6. Pretty poor ____ 7. Very poor
3. How much progress do you feel your client made in dealing with his/her problems in this session?	____ 1. A great deal of progress ____ 2. Considerable progress ____ 3. Moderate progress ____ 4. Some progress ____ 5. A little progress ____ 6. Didn't get anywhere in this session ____ 7. In some ways my problems have gotten worse this session
4. In this session something shifted for my client. S/he saw something differently or experienced something freshly:	____ 1. Not at all ____ 2. Very slightly ____ 3. Slightly ____ 4. Somewhat ____ 5. Moderately ____ 6. Considerably ____ 7. Very much

III. Client Modes of Engagement

Please rate the extent to which your client was engaging in each of the following modes of engagement during the session:

Absent	Occasional (1 – 5% of responses)	Common (10 – 20% of responses)	Frequent (25 – 45% of responses)	Extensive (≥ 50% of responses)
1	2	3	4	5

1 2 3 4 5	1. <u>Flooded</u>: Overwhelmed by unsymbolized emotion; disorganized and chaotic, with various other elements present in a disorganized fashion
1 2 3 4 5	2. <u>Distanced/Dissociated</u>: Avoiding or holding painful or frightening feelings or experiences at bay
1 2 3 4 5	3. <u>Externalized</u>: Attending exclusively to other people, external events; may be specific or general
1 2 3 4 5	4. <u>Somatizing</u>: Attending exclusively to chronic pain or illness signs
1 2 3 4 5	5. <u>Abstract/Purely conceptual</u>: Formulating things in linguistic or abstract terms without reference to concrete experiencing
1 2 3 4 5	6. <u>Impulsive</u>: Focused purely on wishes or actions; acting out; driven, without reflection
1 2 3 4 5	7. <u>Externally attending</u>: Mindful receptive focus on perceptual experience/memories; emotionally engaged narrative
1 2 3 4 5	8. <u>Body-focused</u>: Careful attention to bodily experience and felt meaning
1 2 3 4 5	9. <u>Emotion-focused</u>: Awareness and symbolization of immediate emotional experience
1 2 3 4 5	10. <u>Reflexive-symbolizing</u>: Active curiosity and reflection on the meaning, value or understanding of experience
1 2 3 4 5	11. <u>Active expression</u>: expressing wants/needs; enacting strong emotions
1 2 3 4 5	12. <u>Re-perceiving/Altered perception</u>: Noticing new things not attended to before or seeing previously-attended-to things in a different light; new understanding, insight or awareness
1 2 3 4 5	13. <u>Body-shift/Relief</u>: Allowing oneself to enjoy the easing of previous problem-related tension carried in the body
1 2 3 4 5	14. <u>Receiving emotional change</u>: Allowing oneself to feel new, more adaptive emotions
1 2 3 4 5	15. <u>Self-reflection/Meaning perspective</u>: Standing back from successfully processed experiencing; becoming dis-embedded from previous assumptions so as to appreciate new possibilities, achieving a new explanation of one's situation or feelings
1 2 3 4 5	16. <u>Action-planning</u>: Moving towards action on the basis of successfully processed experiencing; problem-solving; oriented towards developing productive solutions

IV. EFT Therapy Principles

Please rate how well you feel you applied each of the treatment principles below, using this rating scale:

1	Much improvement in application needed: I felt like a beginner, as if I didn't have the concept.
2	Moderate improvement needed: I felt like an advanced beginner, who is beginning to do this, but needs to work on the concept more.
3	Slight improvement in application needed: I need to make a focused effort to do more of this.
4	Adequate application of principle: I did enough of this, but need to keep working on improving how well I do it.
5	Good application of principle: I did enough of this and did it skilfully.
6	Excellent application of principle: I did this consistently and even applied it in a creative way.

1 2 3 4 5 6	1. I was <u>empathically attuned</u> to the client's experiencing (by letting go of presumptions, entering the client's world, resonating from my own experience, sorting through variety, grasping what is important and readjusting understandings as experiencing evolves).
1 2 3 4 5 6	2. I expressed <u>empathy</u>/understanding, <u>presence</u>/genuineness, and <u>prizing</u>/caring to my client.
1 2 3 4 5 6	3. I facilitated client–therapist <u>collaboration</u> and mutual involvement in goals and tasks of therapy, through experiential teaching, goal/task identification and negotiation.
1 2 3 4 5 6	4. I attended and <u>responded carefully and differentially</u> to important client processes (tasks, steps within tasks, client micro-processes and emotion processing modes) at different times in the session.
1 2 3 4 5 6	5. I helped client use key therapeutic tasks to move themselves from problematic to adaptive emotions through an <u>emotional deepening process</u>.
1 2 3 4 5 6	6. I facilitated client <u>self-development</u>, new emotional meaning, and a sense of personal agency and forward movement in life.

V. Task Resolution and Intervention Scales

<u>Instructions</u>. For each therapeutic task on the following pages, rate each of the following using the scales provided:

<u>Resolution Scales</u>: Rate how far the client got on each therapeutic task, regardless of therapist task intervention; circle the furthest point reached on the scale.

<u>Presence Rating Scale</u>: Use this scale to rate the extent to which you attempted to engage the client in each of the therapeutic task activities listed below.

<u>Quality Rating Scale</u>: Use this scale to rate how well or skilfully you think you facilitated (vs. interfered) with each of the therapeutic tasks listed.

Note that tasks may overlap; it is possible to work on two tasks at the same time (e.g., Empathic Exploration and Focusing or Two chair dialogue; Empathic Prizing and Meaning Creation).

1. Developing and Maintaining a Safe Working Alliance

    A. Rate current level of client working alliance

0	Client drops out of therapy or announces decision to stop because of alliance problems.
1	Client physically present but safe, working environment not yet achieved.
2	Work on trust/bond: Begins therapy, but worried that therapist will misunderstand, judge, or be insincere, intrusive or untrustworthy.
3	Work on therapeutic focus: Trusts therapist and begins to engage in therapy process, but has difficulty finding and maintaining a focus, is scattered or generally defers to therapist.
4	Work on goal agreement: Therapeutic focus located but ambivalent about change, not firmly committed to working towards goals related to main therapeutic focus; sees the causes of his/her problems differently from therapist.
5	Work on task agreement: Committed to change, but has difficulty turning attention inward; questions the purpose and value of working with emotions/experiencing; has expectations about tasks and process that diverge from those of therapist.
6	Productive working environment: Client trusts therapist, engages actively in productive therapeutic work.

    B. Task Intervention: Facilitate alliance formation through meta-communication, demonstration of caring, empathy; negotiation of therapeutic focus, goals, and tasks.

PRESENCE		QUALITY	
1	Clearly absent	1	Significant interference with task
2	Possibly present	2	Moderate interference
3	Present but brief	3	Slight interference; more needed/missed marker
4	Present, moderate length	4	Neutral; not applicable
5	Present, extended in length	5	Slightly skilful facilitation
		6	Moderately skilful facilitation
		7	Excellent facilitation of task

2. Relationship Dialogue for Repair of Alliance Difficulties

    A. Client Task Resolution

0	Marker absent (therapeutic work proceeds without difficulty).
1	Marker: Implies or mentions complaint or dissatisfaction about nature or progress of therapy, or therapeutic relationship. (Withdrawal: disengages from process; Confrontation: challenges, questions therapy.) Describe: _____
2	Accepts task, presents complaint or dissatisfaction directly or in more detail. (Withdrawal difficulty: Admits to difficulty.)
3	Explores nature, possible joint sources of complaint/dissatisfaction/difficulty; seeks both to understand therapist side and to elaborate, understand own part in difficulty.
4	Develops, describes shared understanding of source of difficulty.
5	Reaches a new view of general nature or mutual roles in therapy; explores practical solutions with therapist.
6	Expresses genuine satisfaction or obvious renewed enthusiasm for therapy.

     B.   Task Intervention: Raise and facilitate mutual dialogue about difficulty.

PRESENCE		QUALITY	
1	Clearly absent	1	Significant interference with task
2	Possibly present	2	Moderate interference
3	Present but brief	3	Slight interference; more needed/missed marker
4	Present, moderate length	4	Neutral; not applicable
5	Present, extended in length	5	Slightly skilful facilitation
		6	Moderately skilful facilitation
		7	Excellent facilitation of task

3.   Clearing a Space for Attentional Focus Difficulty

     A.   Client Task Resolution

0	Marker absent
1	Marker: Attentional Focus Difficulty: Reports or evidences being stuck, overwhelmed, or blank.
2	Attends to internal 'problem space.'
3	Lists concerns or problematic experiences.
4	Sets concerns or problems aside; uses imagination to contain or create psychological distance from problems, may identify most important concern to work on.
5	Appreciates cleared internal space; enjoys relief, sense of free or safe internal space.
6	Generalizes cleared space; develops general appreciation for need, value or possibility of clear/safe space in his/her life.

B. Task Intervention: Helps client clear an imagined internal/bodily space, list, set aside problems; helps client appreciate cleared space or identify concern to work on.

PRESENCE	QUALITY
1 Clearly absent	1 Significant interference with task
2 Possibly present	2 Moderate interference
3 Present but brief	3 Slight interference; more needed/missed marker
4 Present, moderate length	4 Neutral; not applicable
5 Present, extended in length	5 Slightly skilful facilitation
	6 Moderately skilful facilitation
	7 Excellent facilitation of task

4. Experiential Focusing for an Unclear Feeling

   A. Client Task Resolution

0 Marker absent
1 Marker: Unclear feeling: Presents or confirms vague/nagging concern, or discusses concerns in global, abstract, superficial or externalized (circle one) manner.
2 Attends to the unclear concern, including whole feeling.
3 Searches for potential descriptions (felt quality words, images) for unclear feeling; checks descriptions for accuracy (without feeling shift).
4 Feeling shift: Explores labelled feeling more deeply, until bodily sense of discomfort eases and experienced lack of clarity disappears.
5 Receives feeling shift: Stays with, appreciates, consolidates feeling shift; keeps self-criticism at bay.
6 Carrying forward: Develops new in-session task, explores implications for change outside of therapy.

B. Task Intervention: Encourages focusing attitude, search for label/handle, exploration of labelled feeling, receiving of feeling shift, and carrying forward.

PRESENCE	QUALITY
1 Clearly absent	1 Significant interference with task
2 Possibly present	2 Moderate interference
3 Present but brief	3 Slight interference; more needed/missed marker
4 Present, moderate length	4 Neutral; not applicable
5 Present, extended in length	5 Slightly skilful facilitation
	6 Moderately skilful facilitation
	7 Excellent facilitation of task

5.   Facilitating Expression of Feelings with Emotional Expression Difficulties

   A.   Client Task Resolution

-	(No zero point)
1	Pre-reflective reaction to situation without awareness; emotion blocked from awareness ('I have no feelings.').
2	Limited conscious awareness of emotion ('I'm not sure if I'm feeling something.').
3	Unclear feeling ('I don't know what I'm feeling.'); or prepackaged description ('I know what I'm feeling without having to check.').
4	Negative attitude towards emotion ('Feelings are dangerous or irrelevant.').
5	Difficulty with appropriate level of emotional expression to therapist/others: Excessive or premature disclosure ('I've told you too much about myself already!'); or perception of therapist/others as unreceptive ('You can't be interested in what I'm feeling.').
6	Successful, appropriate expression of emotion to therapist/significant others.

   B.   Task Intervention: Encourages emotional expression with appropriate response modes, tasks (e.g., evocative/exploratory response, Focusing, Empathic Exploration, Chairwork).

PRESENCE		QUALITY	
1	Clearly absent	1	Significant interference with task
2	Possibly present	2	Moderate interference
3	Present but brief	3	Slight interference; more needed/missed marker
4	Present, moderate length	4	Neutral; not applicable
5	Present, extended in length	5	Slightly skilful facilitation
		6	Moderately skilful facilitation
		7	Excellent facilitation of task

6.   Empathic Affirmation of Vulnerability

   A.   Client Task Resolution

0	Marker absent
1	Marker: Mentions strong negative self-related feeling and expresses distress about it; describe form of vulnerability: _____
2	Describes deeper feelings in response to therapist's empathic affirmation.
3	Expresses more intense vulnerability.
4	Seems to touch bottom; expresses dreaded emotion or painful aspect of self in full intensity.
5	Describes or expresses reduced distress, greater calmness.
6	Expresses sense of self as whole, acceptable or capable.

B. Task Intervention: Provides genuine, empathic, affirming presence as client descends into dreaded vulnerability, then supports re-emergent client growth-oriented experiencing.

PRESENCE	QUALITY
1 Clearly absent	1 Significant interference with task
2 Possibly present	2 Moderate interference
3 Present but brief	3 Slight interference; more needed/missed marker
4 Present, moderate length	4 Neutral; not applicable
5 Present, extended in length	5 Slightly skilful facilitation
	6 Moderately skilful facilitation
	7 Excellent facilitation of task

7. Narrative Retelling of a Traumatic/Painful Experience (non-PRP)

A. Client Task Resolution

0	Marker absent (abstract, superficial or prepackaged descriptions of an event/experience).
1	Marker present: Refers to a traumatic/painful experience about which a story could be told (e.g., traumatic event, disrupted life story, nightmare). Nature of experience:
	_____
2	Elaboration; begins detailed, concrete or factual narrative of particular event/experience; describes what happened from external or logical point of view.
3	Dwells on important moments or aspects of trauma, re-experiences parts of it in session.
4	Differentiates personal, idiosyncratic, newly emerged meanings of the experience from an internal point of view.
5	Thoughtfully weighs and tentatively evaluates alternative, differentiated views of the experience.
6	Integrates previously unconnected or inconsistent aspects of the experience; expresses broader or more integrated view of self, others or world.

B. Task Intervention: Facilitate client re-telling/re-experiencing through unfolding and exploration process.

PRESENCE	QUALITY
1 Clearly absent	1 Significant interference with task
2 Possibly present	2 Moderate interference
3 Present but brief	3 Slight interference; more needed/missed marker
4 Present, moderate length	4 Neutral; not applicable

5	Present, extended in length	5	Slightly skilful facilitation
		6	Moderately skilful facilitation
		7	Excellent facilitation of task

8.   Unfolding Problematic Reactions

A.   Client Task Resolution

0	Marker absent
1	Marker: Describes unexpected, puzzling personal reaction (Circle: behaviour, emotion reaction). Describe: _____
2	'Re-enters' the scene, recalls and re-experiences the time when the reaction was triggered.
3	Recalls salient aspects of stimulus situation. Explores both own internal affective reaction to situation and own subjective construal of potential impact of stimulus situation.
4	Reaches 'meaning bridge.' Discovers link between problematic reaction and own construal of potential impact of stimulus situation.
5	Recognizes this as example of broader aspect of own mode of functioning that is interfering with personal needs, wants, views, or values.
6	Full resolution: Develops broad new view of important aspects of own mode of functioning and what self-changes to make. Begins to feel empowered to make change(s).

B.   Task Intervention: Systematic evocative unfolding: helps client to review in detail perceptions and emotions involved in problematic reaction; helps client to explore broader implications.

PRESENCE	QUALITY
1 Clearly absent	1 Significant interference with task
2 Possibly present	2 Moderate interference
3 Present but brief	3 Slight interference; more needed/missed marker
4 Present, moderate length	4 Neutral; not applicable
5 Present, extended in length	5 Slightly skilful facilitation
	6 Moderately skilful facilitation
	7 Excellent facilitation of task

9.   Creation of Meaning for Meaning Protest

A.   Client Task Resolution

0	Marker absent (emotional arousal with vagueness or confusion).
1	Marker: Describes an experience discrepant with cherished belief; in an emotionally aroused state. (Life event: _____; Cherished belief: _____)
2	Clarifies, specifies nature of cherished belief and emotional reactions to challenging life event.
3	Searches for origins of cherished belief; develops hypothesis.
4	Evaluates and judges continued tenability of cherished belief (in relation to present experience); expresses desire to alter cherished belief.
5	Revision: Alters or eliminates cherished belief.
6	Describes nature of change needed or develops plans for future.

    B.   Task Intervention: Facilitates client meaning work; helps client to symbolize felt meaning of painful life event and describe and ultimately re-examine challenged cherished belief(s).

PRESENCE		QUALITY	
1	Clearly absent	1	Significant interference with task
2	Possibly present	2	Moderate interference
3	Present but brief	3	Slight interference; more needed/missed marker
4	Present, moderate length	4	Neutral; not applicable
5	Present, extended in length	5	Slightly skilful facilitation
		6	Moderately skilful facilitation
		7	Excellent facilitation of task

10. Two Chair Work for Conflict Splits

    A.   Client Task Resolution

0	Marker absent
1	Marker: Describes split in which one aspect of self is critical of, or coercive towards, another aspect. Describe two aspects and circle type: self-criticism, self-coaching, self-interruption, attributed, depression, anxiety, motivational, toxic: _____).
2	Clearly expresses criticisms, expectations, or 'shoulds' to self in concrete, specific manner.
3	Primary underlying feelings/needs begin to emerge in response to the criticisms. Critic differentiates values/standards. Experiencer may collapse/recover.
4	Clearly expresses needs and wants associated with a newly experienced feeling.
5	Genuinely accepts own feelings and needs. May show compassion, concern, and respect for self.
6	Clear understanding of how various feelings, needs, and wishes may be accommodated and how previously antagonistic sides of self may be reconciled.

B. Task Intervention: Facilitates client dialogue between conflicting aspects of self.

PRESENCE	QUALITY
1 Clearly absent	1 Significant interference with task
2 Possibly present	2 Moderate interference
3 Present but brief	3 Slight interference; more needed/missed marker
4 Present, moderate length	4 Neutral; not applicable
5 Present, extended in length	5 Slightly skilful facilitation
	6 Moderately skilful facilitation
	7 Excellent facilitation of task

11. Empty Chair Work for Unfinished Business

A. Client Task Resolution

0	Marker absent
1	Marker: Blames, complains or expresses hurt or longing in relation to a significant Other. (person: _____)
2	Speaks to imagined Other and expresses unresolved feelings (e.g., resentment, hurt).
3	Differentiates complaint into underlying feeling; experiences and expresses relevant emotions (e.g., sadness, anger) with a high degree of emotional arousal.
4	Experiences unmet need(s) as valid and expresses them assertively.
5	Comes to understand and see Other in a new way, either in a more positive light or as a less powerful person who has/had problems of his/her own.
6	Affirms Self and lets go of unresolved feeling, either by forgiving Other or holding Other accountable.

B. Task Intervention: Helps client express unresolved hurt, anger, unmet needs to imagined Other; may help client enact role of the Other.

PRESENCE	QUALITY
1 Clearly absent	1 Significant interference with task
2 Possibly present	2 Moderate interference
3 Present but brief	3 Slight interference; more needed/missed marker
4 Present, moderate length	4 Neutral; not applicable
5 Present, extended in length	5 Slightly skilful facilitation
	6 Moderately skilful facilitation
	7 Excellent facilitation of task

12. Compassionate Self-soothing for Stuck Emotional Suffering

   A. Client Task Resolution

0	Marker absent
1	Marker: Expresses pain/anguish with hopelessness or insecurity (stuck, collapsed self-state).
2	Evokes sad/scared/collapsed self-aspect or Other. Identifies appropriate self–Other combination: _____
3	Enact compassionate self-aspect or Other.
4	Experiences emotional/bodily relief.
5	Shifts towards more positive, empowered view of self.
6	Considers how to extend this process in their life.

   B. Task Intervention: Helps client in Compassionate Person role to comfort or affirm stuck/suffering aspect.

PRESENCE		QUALITY	
1	Clearly absent	1	Significant interference with task
2	Possibly present	2	Moderate interference
3	Present but brief	3	Slight interference; more needed/missed marker
4	Present, moderate length	4	Neutral; not applicable
5	Present, extended in length	5	Slightly skilful facilitation
		6	Moderately skilful facilitation
		7	Excellent facilitation of task

VI. EFT Response Modes

Use this scale to rate the degree to which each of the items below was present in this session:

Absent	Occasional (1 – 5% of responses)	Common (10 – 20% of responses)	Frequent (25 – 45% of responses)	Extensive (≥ 50% of responses)
1	2	3	4	5

1 2 3 4 5	1.	**Personal Disclosure**: Share relevant information about self as a person, outside session.
1 2 3 4 5	2.	**Process Disclosure**: Share own here-and-now reactions, intentions or limitations.

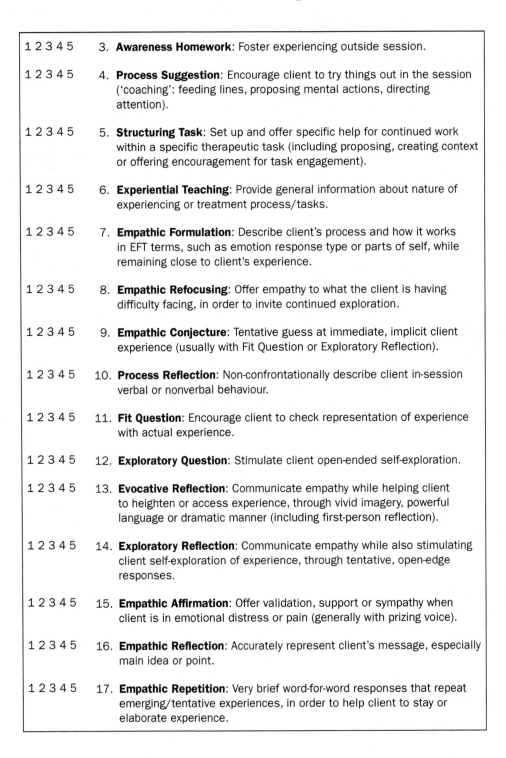

1 2 3 4 5   3. **Awareness Homework**: Foster experiencing outside session.

1 2 3 4 5   4. **Process Suggestion**: Encourage client to try things out in the session ('coaching': feeding lines, proposing mental actions, directing attention).

1 2 3 4 5   5. **Structuring Task**: Set up and offer specific help for continued work within a specific therapeutic task (including proposing, creating context or offering encouragement for task engagement).

1 2 3 4 5   6. **Experiential Teaching**: Provide general information about nature of experiencing or treatment process/tasks.

1 2 3 4 5   7. **Empathic Formulation**: Describe client's process and how it works in EFT terms, such as emotion response type or parts of self, while remaining close to client's experience.

1 2 3 4 5   8. **Empathic Refocusing**: Offer empathy to what the client is having difficulty facing, in order to invite continued exploration.

1 2 3 4 5   9. **Empathic Conjecture**: Tentative guess at immediate, implicit client experience (usually with Fit Question or Exploratory Reflection).

1 2 3 4 5   10. **Process Reflection**: Non-confrontationally describe client in-session verbal or nonverbal behaviour.

1 2 3 4 5   11. **Fit Question**: Encourage client to check representation of experience with actual experience.

1 2 3 4 5   12. **Exploratory Question**: Stimulate client open-ended self-exploration.

1 2 3 4 5   13. **Evocative Reflection**: Communicate empathy while helping client to heighten or access experience, through vivid imagery, powerful language or dramatic manner (including first-person reflection).

1 2 3 4 5   14. **Exploratory Reflection**: Communicate empathy while also stimulating client self-exploration of experience, through tentative, open-edge responses.

1 2 3 4 5   15. **Empathic Affirmation**: Offer validation, support or sympathy when client is in emotional distress or pain (generally with prizing voice).

1 2 3 4 5   16. **Empathic Reflection**: Accurately represent client's message, especially main idea or point.

1 2 3 4 5   17. **Empathic Repetition**: Very brief word-for-word responses that repeat emerging/tentative experiences, in order to help client to stay or elaborate experience.

VII. Content Directive Interventions

Use this scale to rate the following items:

Clearly Absent	Possibly present	Present but very brief and 'in-mode' (e.g., tentative, in answer to question)	Present, brief, in 'expert' manner	Present, extended, 'expert' manner
1	2	3	4	5

1 2 3 4 5	1. **Give News**: Responses intended to tell the client something new about self or others (i.e., interpretations). Describe:
1 2 3 4 5	2. **Offer Solutions**: Responses intended to modify client behaviour with regard to presented problems (i.e., general advisements). Describe:
1 2 3 4 5	3. **Offer Expert Reassurance**: Responses directly intended to make the client feel good or less bad, given from an 'expert' position. Describe:
1 2 3 4 5	4. **Disagree/Confront**: Responses intended to correct, criticize or point out discrepancies. Describe:
1 2 3 4 5	5. **Nonexperiential Task/Content Direction**: e.g., introduce new subject/task such as problem-solving or client analysis of third parties. Describe:
1 2 3 4 5	6. **Purely informational questions**: Gather specific information without encouraging exploration. Describe:

Appendix 2

Person-Centred & Experiential Psychotherapy Scale – EFT-T Supplement (Draft Therapist Version 1.0, 29/10/18)

Client ID:	Session:
Rater:	Segment:

EFT-1. Empathic Attunement

How well did I express empathic attunement to the client?

Did my responses convey an active, accurate and consistent understanding of the client's inner experiences as these evolve from moment to moment in the session? Or conversely, did my responses fail to track important experiences of the client? Empathic attunement is expressed by the use of voice quality that mirrors the emotional tone of the client or conveys prizing or affirmation. It can be conveyed by a range of empathic responses focusing on the client's inner perspective:

- *Empathic reflections, which accurately represent most important main aspect of the client's message or communicated experience.*
- *Empathic repetitions, which briefly repeat key words or phrases from the client to show tracking.*
- *Empathic affirmations, which express validation, support or caring if the client is in emotional distress or pain, using both words and prizing vocal tone.*
- *Exploratory reflections, which communicate empathy and encourage client self-exploration through tentative, open-edge or growth-oriented responses and use voice quality that expresses curiosity and interest.*
- *Evocative reflections, which communicate empathy while helping the client to heighten or activate experience, through vivid imagery, powerful language or dramatic manner (including speaking in the first person as if the client or using evocative, expressive voice quality).*

- *Process reflections, which non-confrontationally describe the client's in-session verbal or nonverbal behaviour.*
- *Empathic conjectures, which tentatively guess at immediate, implicit or unexpressed client experiences. (Best if delivered in a respectful, exploratory manner that encourages the client to check inside whether the conjecture fits.)*
- *Empathic formulations, which describe the client's specific difficulties in theory terms, such as parts of the self, emotional avoidance or conditions of worth.*
- *Empathic refocusing responses, which offer empathy to what the client is having difficulty facing, in order to gently invite continued exploration.*
- *Attunement to client nonverbal behaviour, including mirroring of client posture and facial expression.*

---

1   **Much improvement in application needed:** I acted like a beginner, as if I didn't really have the concept of empathic attunement or empathic communication; I did not use an appropriate voice quality.

2   **Moderate improvement needed:** I acted like an advanced beginner, who is beginning to empathically attune to the client but who really needs to work on communicating it more and better. I tried to adapt the voice quality to the therapeutic process.

3   **Slight improvement in empathic attunement, communication and voice quality needed:** I need to make a focused effort to do better with my empathic attunement, including communicating it and adapting my voice quality more and better.

4   **Adequate empathic attunement, communication and voice quality:** I did enough empathic attunement and communication but need to keep working on improving how well I do it, such as supporting it with unconditional positive regard and genuine presence.

5   **Good empathic attunement, communication and voice quality:** I did enough of this and did it skilfully, offering it in a genuine, present, and unconditionally caring manner.

6   **Excellent empathic attunement, communication and voice quality:** I did this consistently, to some depth and even carried it out in a creative, carefully nuanced way.

EFT-2. Marker Identification

How well did my responses accurately pick up on key client task markers for what the client wanted to work on in the session?

Markers are observable indicators that the client is ready to work on certain therapeutic tasks. This includes accurately identifying the most important marker(s) and confirming them with the client. Accurate marker identification is 'task empathy' for the client's personal agency, that is, how they want to use the session.

Circle any of the following markers that you accurately picked up on; cross out any that were present that you missed:

- *Vulnerability (painful feelings): Empathic affirmation*
- *Unclear feeling (vague, external or absent), unclear or absent felt sense: Focusing*
- *Problematic reaction point (puzzling overreaction to specific situation): Systematic evocative unfolding*
- *Conflict splits (self-critical, self-interruptive, self-coaching): Two chair work (Two Chair Dialogue or Enactment)*
- *Unfinished business (lingering): Empty chair work*
- *Anguish/emotional suffering: Compassionate self-soothing*
- *Attention problems/overwhelmed: Space clearing*
- *Alliance difficulties: Alliance Dialogue*

---

1   **No markers identified:** Clear client markers were present but I consistently missed them, and in fact failed to convey any sense of the client as a personal agent with their own agenda or goals for the session.

2   **Most markers missed or imposed own tasks on client:** I had the concept of markers to a certain extent but missed most of those offered by my client in this session. Alternatively, I imposed tasks I thought were important on the client in the absence of appropriate markers.

3   **Key markers missed:** I picked up on some markers but missed key ones.

4   **Key markers picked up:** I picked up key markers for work with my client but fed them back to my client in an awkward manner.

5   **Key markers differentiated and offered back in a skilful manner:** I picked up key markers and accurately formulated them back to my client in a differentiated manner (e.g., I accurately reflected back to my client the precise type of conflict split they presented).

6   **Unusual or new markers creatively and sensitively picked up and offered:** I picked up and reflected back key client markers consistently, sensitively, and even creatively.

EFT-3. Emotion Deepening

How well did I help my client deepen their emotional experience?

How skilfully and sensitively did I facilitate the client in the process of deepening their emotion experiencing?

This often involves the use of appropriate therapeutic tasks but more importantly can be seen in the therapist's close empathic tracking and skilful use of deepening exploratory questions and empathic conjectures. It can be helpful to assess how well you helped the client move through the following sequence:

- *Global distress (undifferentiated emotions)*
- *Secondary reactive emotional responses (often emotions associated with presenting problems or symptoms)*
- *Primary maladaptive emotional responses (old familiar stuck emotions)*
- *Core pain (the most central or important primary maladaptive emotions)*

- *Unmet needs associated with core pain*
- *Primary adaptive emotional responses (differentiated emotions, primary hurt/grief, assertive anger, self-compassion)*

---

1 **Emotion deepening completely absent:** I consistently missed opportunities to help my client to deepen their emotional experiences, and instead generally offered responses that moved the client away from their feelings and towards more external or less differentiated experiences.

2 **Mostly flattening responses:** I often missed opportunities to deepen the client's emotions and mostly responded in a more external/less differentiated manner.

3 **Deepening responses present but poorly done:** I offered opportunities to help my client to deepen, but these were quite awkward and were imposed on my client, thus generally interfered with my client's process.

4 **Deepening responses clearly present but inconsistent or awkward:** I offered deepening responses at key moments but was inconsistent and at times somewhat awkward.

5 **Deepening responses consistent and skilful:** I consistently and skilfully took opportunities to help my client to deepen their emotional experiences, helping them move from global distress towards core pain.

6 **Emotional deepening offered in a highly attuned and creative manner:** I sensitively and artfully facilitated my client's emotional deepening, including skilfully working with their ambivalence about deepening.

EFT-4. Appropriate Use of EFT Tasks

How well did I carry out appropriate EFT tasks?

Having accurately identified one or more appropriate tasks, how skilfully and sensitively did I facilitate my client through the stages of these tasks, including:

- *Introducing and setting up the task*
- *Helping my client to enter into the task in order to evoke experience*
- *Staying with the key processes in the task where appropriate*
- *Picking up emerging shifts or new experiences*
- *Shifting to a different or emerging task where appropriate*
- *Coming to closure if the time runs out for further work on the task*
- *Helping my client to stay with and develop a meaning perspective on any new experiences that might have emerged*
- *Tasks:*
  - o *Empathic affirmation*
  - o *Experiential focusing*
  - o *Systematic evocative unfolding*

      o   *Two chair work (Two chair dialogue or enactment)*
      o   *Empty chair work*
      o   *Compassionate self-soothing*
      o   *Clearing space*

---

1   **Avoided even obvious tasks**: I failed to carry out EFT tasks even when the markers were obvious and pressing.

2   **Imposed task on client in an insensitive, mechanical or intrusive manner**: I imposed the wrong task on my client, or carried it out in a quite intrusive, insensitive or mechanical manner.

3   **Offered an appropriate task but in a clumsy, awkward manner that blocked client**: I offered an appropriate task but did so in a generally wooden, awkward or clumsy manner that blocked the client's process.

4   **Generally skilful in facilitating client work on task, but occasional minor awkwardness or missed opportunities**: My facilitation of my client's movement through tasks was generally adequate, even though there were minor problems, such as missed opportunities to deepen or occasional minor awkwardness in facilitation.

5   **Task facilitation was consistent and skilful**: I was fully immersed in the task with my client, consistently and skilfully offering client opportunities to use the task to deepen their emotional experience and to progress through it towards resolution.

6   **Facilitated client work on tasks in a highly attuned and creative manner**: I was deeply and exquisitely attuned to the client in their shared work on the task, responding in creative ways, such as appropriately implementing the task in a novel manner or skilfully helping the client to navigate difficult blocks, such as ambivalence or emotional avoidance.

EFT-5. EFT Case Formulation: Ability to Think about Clients in EFT Terms

How skilful was I in thinking about my client in EFT terms and using this to facilitate our relationship and the therapeutic work?

EFT case formulation takes various forms and can be seen in a variety of ways:

- *Offering explicit empathic formulation responses that simply label aspects of self, emotion response types or markers*
- *Collaboratively constructing with the client more complex narratives that involve sequences of processes (e.g., negative interpersonal cycle formulations in couples work)*
- *Giving responses that imply case formulations by orienting to key client processes, such as markers, aspects of self, types of emotion response, emotion dysregulation*

A skilful EFT case formulation is collaborative, exploratory, accurate, friendly and specific, as opposed to imposed, definite, patronising/critical or generic.

1   **Intrusive, pejorative or non-EFT case formulations**: I imposed inaccurate or unwanted case formulations on my client, ignoring their objections; my case formulations patronised or pathologized my client, potentially damaging their sense of self; I persistently elaborated non-EFT case formulations (e.g., CBT or psychodynamic).

2   **No case formulation**: I offered no empathic formulation responses and made no apparent reference or response to any EFT concepts or case formulation elements, including markers, aspects of self, emotion responses types, and modes of engagement.

3   **Awkward, inaccurate EFT case formulations**: My case formulations were recognizably EFT in their content but were generally inaccurate or were delivered in an awkward manner that interfered with the client's process.

4   **Adequate EFT case formulation**: I offered EFT case formulations that were generally, although not always, accurate, collaborative, exploratory, and specific. (There may be occasional minor inaccuracies, overly generic elements or awkwardness.)

5   **Good EFT case formulation**: I consistently provided EFT case formulation elements that were collaborative, exploratory, accurate, friendly, and specific, in such a way that even minor inaccuracies were quickly left behind without distracting my client.

6   **Excellent EFT case formulation**: Working in deep collaboration with my client, I artfully built up shared, unique EFT case formulations in an exploratory process that affirmed my client and provided them with a clear way forward in therapy.

Appendix 3

Helpful Aspects of Therapy Form (HAT) (Version 3.2, 05/2008)

1. Of the events which occurred in this session, which one do you feel was the most **important** or **helpful** for you personally? (By 'event' we mean something that happened in the session. It might be something you said or did, or something your therapist or counsellor said or did.)

2. Please describe what made this event important/helpful and what you got out of it.

3. How **helpful or hindering** was this particular **event**? Rate it on the following scale.

(Put an 'X' at the appropriate point; half-point ratings are OK; e.g., 7.5.)

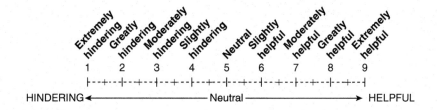

4. About where in the session did this event occur?

5. About how long did the event last?

6. Did anything else particularly **helpful** happen during this session?
   YES   NO

   a. If yes, please rate how **helpful** this event was:

   Slightly ☐6   Moderately ☐7   Greatly ☐8   Extremely ☐9

   b. Please describe the event briefly:

7. Did anything happen during the session which might have been **hindering**?

   YES   NO

   a. If yes, please rate how **hindering** the event was:

   Slightly ☐4   Moderately ☐3   Greatly ☐2   Extremely ☐1

   b. Please describe this event briefly:

References

Angus, L., & Greenberg, L. (2011). *Working with narrative in emotion-focused therapy*. Washington, DC: American Psychological Association.

Barge, A., & Elliott, R. (2016). Clients' experiences of ending person-centred/experiential time limited therapy. Unpublished manuscript, Counselling Unit, University of Strathclyde, Glasgow, Scotland. Available at: www.dropbox.com/s/ghddw0ksv3g6fjl/_Barge%20%26%20Elliott%20Endings%202016.docx?dl=0

Barkham, M., Margison, F., Leach, C., Lucock, M., Mellor-Clark, J., Evans, C., Benson, L., Connell, J., Audin, K., & McGrath, G. (2001). Service profiling and outcomes benchmarking using the CORE-OM: Toward practice-based evidence in the psychological therapies. *Journal of Consulting and Clinical Psychology, 69*, 184–196.

Baucom, D. H., Shoham, V., Mueser, K. T., Daiuto, A. D., & Stickle, T. R. (1998). Empirically supported couple and family interventions for marital distress and adult mental health problems. *Journal of Consulting and Clinical Psychology, 66*(1), 53–88.

Bolger, E. A. (1999). Grounded theory analysis of emotional pain. *Psychotherapy Research, 9*, 342–362.

Bordin, E. S. (1979). The generalizability of the psychoanalytic concept of working alliance. *Psychotherapy: Theory, Research and Practice, 16*, 252–260.

Brodley, B. T. (1990). Client-centered and experiential: Two different therapies. In G. Lietaer, J. Rombauts, & R. Van Balen (Eds.), *Client-centered and experiential psychotherapy towards the nineties* (pp. 87–107). Leuven, Belgium: Leuven University Press.

Bruner, J. (1991). The narrative construction of reality. *Critical Inquiry, 18*, 1–21. DOI: 10.1086/448619

Clarke, K. M. (1989). Creation of meaning: An emotional processing task in psychotherapy. *Psychotherapy, 26*, 139–148.

Clarke, K. M. (1991). A performance model of the creation of meaning event. *Psychotherapy, 28*, 395–401.

Clarke, K. M. (1993). Creation of meaning in incest survivors. *Journal of Cognitive Psychotherapy, 7*, 195–203.

Coates, W. H., White, H. V., & Schapiro, J. S. (1966). *The emergence of liberal humanism: An intellectual history of Western Europe*. New York: McGraw-Hill.

Cornell, A. W. (1996). *The power of focusing*. Oakland, CA: New Harbinger.

Cowie, C. G. (2014). Doing being: Conversation analysis of a good outcome case of person-centred therapy. Unpublished MSc dissertation, University of Strathclyde, Glasgow, Scotland.

Cummings, N., & Sayama, M. (1995). *Focused psychotherapy: A casebook of brief intermittent psychotherapy throughout the life cycle.* Routledge.

Damasio, A. (1999). *The feeling of what happens: Body and emotion in the making of consciousness.* New York: Harcourt.

Decety, J., & Ickes, W. (Eds.) (2009). *The social neuroscience of empathy.* Cambridge, MA: MIT Press.

Decety, J., & Lamm, C. (2009). Empathy versus personal distress: Recent evidence from social neuroscience. In J. Decety & W. Ickes (Eds.) (2009), *The social neuroscience of empathy* (pp. 199–213). Cambridge, MA: MIT Press.

Diamond, G. S., Diamond, G. M., & Levy, S. A. (2014). *Attachment-based family therapy for depressed adolescents.* Washington, DC: American Psychological Association.

Dolhanty, J., & LaFrance, A. (2019). Emotion-focused family therapy for eating disorders. In L. S. Greenberg & R. N. Goldman (Eds.), *Clinical handbook of emotion-focused therapy* (pp. 403–423). Washington, DC: American Psychological Association.

Ekman, P. (1992). An argument for basic emotions. *Cognition & Emotion, 6*(3–4), 169–200. DOI: 10.1080/02699939208411068

Ekman, P., & Davidson, R. J. (Eds.) (1994). *The nature of emotion: Fundamental questions.* Series in affective science. Oxford: Oxford University Press.

Ekman, P., & Friesen, M. V. (1969). The repertoire of nonverbal behavior: Categories, origins, usage and coding. *Semiotica, 1,* 49–98.

Elliott, R. (2016). *Understanding emotion-focused therapy.* [Video]. Counselling Channel (Producer).

Elliott, R. (2019). *EFT Therapist Session Form (ETSF, v6.0).* Unpublished research instrument, Counselling Unit, University of Strathclyde, Glasgow, Scotland.

Elliott, R., Bohart, A. C., Watson, J. C., & Murphy, D. (2018). Therapist empathy and client outcome: An updated meta-analysis. *Psychotherapy, 55,* 399–410. DOI: 10.1037/pst0000175 [supplemental material: http://dx.doi.org/10.1037/pst0000175.supp]

Elliott, R., Clark, C., Wexler, M., Kemeny, V., Brinkerhoff, J., & Mack, C. (1990). The impact of experiential therapy of depression: Initial results. In G. Lietaer, J. Rombauts, & R. Van Balen (Eds.), *Client-centered and experiential psychotherapy in the nineties* (pp. 549–577). Leuven, Belgium: Leuven University Press.

Elliott, R., & Greenberg, L. S. (1997). Multiple voices in process-experiential therapy: Dialogues between aspects of the self. *Journal of Psychotherapy Integration, 7,* 225–239.

Elliott, R., & Greenberg, L. S. (2016). Humanistic-experiential psychotherapy in practice: Emotion-focused therapy. In L. E. Beutler, A. J. Consoli, & B. Bongar (Eds.), *Comprehensive textbook of psychotherapy: Theory and practice* (2nd ed., pp. 106–120). New York: Oxford University Press.

Elliott, R., & MacDonald, J. (2020). Relational dialogue in emotion-focused therapy. *Journal of Clinical Psychology: In Session.* Advance online publication. DOI: 10.1002/jclp.23069

Elliott, R., & Shahar, B. (2019). Emotion-focused therapy for social anxiety. In L. S. Greenberg & R. N. Goldman (Eds.), *Clinical handbook of emotion-focused therapy* (pp. 337–360). Washington, DC: American Psychological Association.

Elliott, R., Sharbanee, J., Watson, J., & Timulak, L. (2019). The outcome of emotion-focused therapy: 2009–2018 meta-analysis update. Paper presented at the meeting of the International Society for Emotion-Focused Therapy, Glasgow, Scotland, August.

Elliott, R., Wagner, J., Sales, C. M. D., Rodgers, B., Alves, P., & Café, M. J. (2016). Psychometrics of the Personal Questionnaire: A client-generated outcome measure. *Psychological Assessment, 28*, 263–278.

Elliott, R., Watson, J., Goldman, R. N., & Greenberg, L. S. (2004). *Learning emotion-focused therapy: The process-experiential approach to change.* Washington, DC: American Psychological Association.

Elliott, R., Watson, J., Greenberg, L. S., Timulak, L., & Freire, E. (2013). Research on humanistic-experiential psychotherapies. In M. J. Lambert (Ed.), *Bergin & Garfield's handbook of psychotherapy and behavior change* (6th ed., pp. 495–538). New York: Wiley.

Elliott, R., Watson, J., Timulak, L., & Sharbanee, J. (in press). Research on humanistic-experiential psychotherapies. In M. Barkham, W. Lutz, & L. Castonguay (Eds.), *Garfield & Bergin's handbook of psychotherapy & behavior change* (7th ed.). New York: Wiley.

Ellison, J. A., Greenberg, L. S., Goldman, R. N., & Angus, L. (2009). Maintenance of gains following experiential therapies for depression. *Journal of Consulting and Clinical Psychology, 77*(1), 103–112. https://doi.org/10.1037/a0014653

Fairbairn, W. R. D. (1952). *Psychoanalytic studies of the personality.* London: Routledge & Kegan Paul.

Foroughe, M., Stillar, A., Goldstein, L., Dolhanty, J., Goodcase, E. T., & LaFrance, A. (2019). Brief emotion-focused family therapy: An intervention for parents of children and adolescents with mental health issues. *Journal of Marital and Family Therapy, 45*, 410–430.

Frankl, V. (1946/2006). *Man's search for meaning.* Boston, MA: Beacon Press.

Freire, E., Elliott, R., & Westwell, G. (2014). Person Centred and Experiential Psychotherapy Scale (PCEPS): Development and reliability of an adherence/competence measure for person-centred and experiential psychotherapies. *Counselling and Psychotherapy Research, 14*, 220–226.

Frick, W. B. (1999). Flight into health: A new interpretation. *Journal of Humanistic Psychology, 39*, 58–81.

Frijda, N. H. (1986). *The emotions.* Cambridge, UK: Cambridge University Press.

Geller, S. M., & Greenberg, L. S. (2012). *Therapeutic presence: A mindful approach to effective psychotherapy.* Washington, DC: American Psychological Association.

Gendlin, E. T. (1981). *Focusing* (2nd ed.). New York: Bantam Books.

Gendron, M., & Barrett, L. F. (2009). Reconstructing the Past: A Century of Ideas About Emotion in Psychology. *Emotion Review, 1*(4), 316–339. doi:10.1177/1754073909338877.

Goetz, J. L., Keltner, D., & Simon-Thomas, E. (2010). Compassion: An evolutionary analysis and empirical review. *Psychological Bulletin, 136*(3), 351–374. https://doi.org/10.1037/a0018807

Goldman, R., & Fox, A. (2010). Self-soothing in emotion-focused therapy: Findings from a task analysis. Paper presented at the conference of the Society for the Exploration of Psychotherapy Integration, Florence, Italy, May.

Goldman, R., & Greenberg, L. S. (2014). *Case formulation in emotion-focused therapy*. Washington, DC: American Psychological Association.

Goldman, R. N., Greenberg, L. S., & Angus, L. (2006). The effects of adding emotion-focused interventions to the client-centered relationship conditions in the treatment of depression. *Psychotherapy Research, 16*, 537–549.

Grant, B. (1990). Principled and instrumental nondirectiveness in person–centered and client-centered therapy. *Person-Centered Review, 5*, 77–88.

Greenberg, L. S. (1984a). A task analysis of intrapersonal conflict resolution. In L. Rice & L. Greenberg (Eds.), *Patterns of change* (pp. 67–123). New York: Guilford Press.

Greenberg, L. S. (1984b). Task analysis: The general approach. In L. Rice & L. Greenberg (Eds.), *Patterns of change* (pp. 124–148). New York: Guilford Press.

Greenberg, L. S. (2002). Termination of experiential therapy. *Journal of Psychotherapy Integration, 12*(3), 358–363.

Greenberg, L. S. (2007). *Emotion-focused therapy over time (Psychotherapy in six sessions)*. [Video]. Washington, DC: American Psychological Association (Producer).

Greenberg, L. S. (2010). Emotion-focused therapy: A clinical synthesis. *Focus: The Journal of Lifelong Learning in Psychiatry, 8*, 32–42.

Greenberg, L. S. (2015). *Emotion-focused therapy: Coaching clients to work through their feelings* (2nd ed.). Washington, DC: American Psychological Association.

Greenberg, L.S. (2020a). *EFT: Working with core emotion*. [Video]. Counselling Channel (Producer).

Greenberg, L.S. (2020b). *EFT: Working with current and historical trauma*. [Video]. Counselling Channel (Producer).

Greenberg, L. S. (in press). *Changing emotion with emotion*. Washington, DC: American Psychological Association.

Greenberg, L. S., & Elliott, R. (1997). Varieties of empathic responding. In A. Bohart & L. S. Greenberg (Eds.), *Empathy reconsidered: New directions in psychotherapy* (pp. 167–186). Washington, DC: American Psychological Association.

Greenberg, L. S., & Goldman, R. N. (2008). *Emotion-focused couples therapy: The dynamics of emotion, love, and power*. Washington, DC: American Psychological Association.

Greenberg, L. S., & Goldman, R. N. (2018). *Clinical handbook of emotion-focused therapy*. Washington, DC: American Psychological Association.

Greenberg, L. S., & Johnson, S. M. (1988). *Emotionally focused therapy for couples*. New York: Guilford Press.

Greenberg, L. S., & Malcolm, W. (2002). Resolving unfinished business: Relating process to outcome. *Journal of Consulting and Clinical Psychology, 70*, 406–416.

Greenberg, L. S., & Paivio, S. (1997). *Working with emotions in psychotherapy*. New York: Guilford Press.

Greenberg, L. S., & Pascual-Leone, J. (1995). A dialectical constructivist approach to experiential change. In R. Neimeyer & M. Mahoney (Eds.), *Constructivism in psychotherapy* (pp. 169–191). Washington, DC: American Psychological Association.

Greenberg, L. S., Rice, L. N., & Elliott, R. (1993). *Facilitating emotional change: The moment-by-moment process.* New York: Guilford Press.

Greenberg, L. S., & Safran, J. D. (1984). Integrating affect and cognition: A perspective on the process of therapeutic change. *Cognitive Therapy & Research, 8,* 559–578.

Greenberg, L. S., & Safran, J. D. (1987). *Emotion in psychotherapy.* New York: Guilford Press.

Greenberg, L. S., & Tomescu, L. R. (2017). *Supervision essentials for emotion-focused therapy.* Washington, DC: American Psychological Association.

Greenberg, L. S., & Warwar, S. H. (2006). Homework in an emotion-focused approach to experiential therapy. *Journal of Psychotherapy Integration, 16*(2), 178–200. https://doi.org/10.1037/1053-0479.16.2.178

Greenberg, L. S., & Watson, J. (1998). Experiential therapy of depression: Differential effects of client-centered relationship conditions and active experiential interventions. *Psychotherapy Research, 8,* 210–224.

Greenberg, L. S., & Watson, J. C. (2005). *Emotion-focused therapy for depression.* Washington, DC: American Psychological Association.

Greenberg, L. S., & Woldarsky Meneses, C. (2019). *Forgiveness and letting go in emotion-focused therapy.* Washington, DC: American Psychological Association.

Grindler Katonah, D. (1999). Clearing a space with someone who has cancer. *Focusing Folio, 18,* 19–26.

Gundrum, M., Lietaer, G., & Van Hees-Matthijssen, C. (1999). Carl Rogers' responses in the 17th session with Miss Mun: Comments from a process-experiential and psychoanalytic perspective. *British Journal of Guidance & Counselling, 27*(4), 461–482.

Hatcher, R. L., & Gillaspy, J. A. (2006). Development and validation of a revised short version of the Working Alliance Inventory. *Psychotherapy Research, 16,* 12–125.

Horvath, A., & Greenberg, L. S. (1989). Development and validation of the Working Alliance Inventory. *Journal of Counseling Psychology, 36,* 223–233.

Ito, M., Greenberg, L. S., Iwakabe, S., & Pascual-Leone, A. (2010). Compassionate emotion regulation: A task analytic approach to studying the process of self-soothing in therapy session. Paper presented at the World Congress of Behavioral and Cognitive Therapies (WCBCT), Boston, MA, June.

Johnson, S. M. (2004). *The practice of emotionally focused marital therapy: Creating connection* (2nd ed.). Philadelphia, PA: Brunner-Mazel.

Johnson, S. M., & Greenberg, L. S. (1985). The differential effects of experiential and problem-solving interventions in resolving marital conflict. *Journal of Consulting and Clinical Psychology, 53,* 313–317.

Johnson, S. M., Hunsley, J., Greenberg, L. S., & Schindler, D. (1999). Emotionally focused couples therapy: Status & challenges. *Journal of Clinical Psychology, 6,* 67–79.

Klein, M. H., Mathieu-Coughlan, P., & Kiesler, D. J. (1986). The experiencing scales. In L. S. Greenberg & W. Pinsof (Eds.), *The psychotherapeutic process* (pp. 21–71). New York: Guilford Press.

LaFrance, A., Henderson, K. A., & Mayman, S. (2019). *Emotion-focused family therapy: A transdiagnostic model for caregiver-focused interventions.* Washington, DC: American Psychological Association.

LeDoux, J. (1996). *The emotional brain: The mysterious underpinnings of emotional life*. New York: Simon & Schuster.

Lewin, K. (1948). *Resolving social conflicts: Selected papers on group dynamics (1935–1946)*. New York: Harper & Brothers.

Lietaer, G. (1993). Authenticity, congruence and transparency. In D. Brazier (Ed.), *Beyond Carl Rogers: Towards a psychotherapy for the 21st century* (pp. 17–46). London: Constable.

Llewelyn, S. (1988). Psychological therapy as viewed by clients and therapists. *British Journal of Clinical Psychology, 27*, 223–238.

Miller, W. R., & Rollnick, S. (2012). *Motivational interviewing: Preparing people for change* (3rd ed.). New York: Guilford Press.

Missirlian, T. M., Toukmanian, S. G., Warwar, S. H., & Greenberg, L. S. (2005). Emotional arousal, client perceptual processing, and the working alliance in experiential psychotherapy for depression. *Journal of Consulting and Clinical Psychology, 73*(5), 861–871.

Moreno, J. L., & Moreno, Z. T. (1959). *Foundations of psychotherapy*. Boston, MA: Beacon Press.

Murphy, D. (2019). *Person-centred experiential counselling for depression* (2nd ed.). London: Sage.

Paivio, S.C. (2013). *Emotion-focused therapy for complex trauma*. [Video]. Washington, DC: American Psychological Association (Producer).

Paivio, S. C., & Pascual-Leone, A. (2010). *Emotion-focused therapy for complex trauma*. Washington, DC: American Psychological Association.

Pascual-Leone, A., & Greenberg, L. S. (2007). Emotional processing in experiential therapy: Why 'the only way out is through'. *Journal of Consulting & Clinical Psychology, 75*, 875–887. DOI: 10.1037/0022-006X.75.6.875

Pascual-Leone, A., & Yeryomenko, N. (2017). The client 'experiencing' scale as a predictor of treatment outcomes: A meta-analysis on psychotherapy process. *Psychotherapy Research, 27*(6), 653–665.

Pennebaker, J. W., & Seagal, J. D. (1999). Forming a story: The health benefits of narrative. *Journal of Clinical Psychology, 55*(10), 1243–1254.

Perls, F. S. (1969). *Gestalt therapy verbatim*. Moab, UT: Real People Press.

Perls, F. S., Hefferline, R. F., & Goodman, P. (1951). *Gestalt therapy*. New York: Julian Press.

Plutchik, R. (1991). *The emotions*. New York: University Press of America.

Portmann, A. (1897/1990). *A zoologist looks at humankind* (trans. J. Schaefer). New York: Columbia University Press.

Pos, A. E., Greenberg, L. S., & Warwar, S. H. (2009). Testing a model of change in the experiential treatment of depression. *Journal of Consulting and Clinical Psychology, 77*(6), 1055–1066.

Prouty, G. (1998). Pre-therapy and pre-symbolic experiencing: Evolutions in person-centered/experiential approaches to psychotic experience. In L. S. Greenberg, J. C. Watson, & G. Lietaer (Eds.), *Handbook of experiential psychotherapy* (pp. 388–409). New York: Guilford Press.

Rice, L. N. (1974). The evocative function of the therapist. In L. N. Rice & D. A. Wexler (Eds.), *Innovations in client-centered therapy* (pp. 289–311). New York: Wiley.

Rice, L. N. (1983). The relationship in client-centered therapy. In M. J. Lambert (Ed.), *Psychotherapy and patient relationships* (pp. 36–60). Homewood, IL: Dow-Jones Irwin.

Rice, L. N., & Greenberg, L. S. (Eds.) (1984). *Patterns of change*. New York: Guilford Press.

Rice, L. N., & Greenberg, L. S. (1991). Two affective change events in client-centered therapy. In J. Safran & L. S. Greenberg (Eds.), *Emotion, psychotherapy and change* (pp. 197–226). New York: Academic Press.

Rice, L. N., & Saperia, E. P. (1984). Task analysis and the resolution of problematic reactions. In L. N. Rice & L. S. Greenberg (Eds.), *Patterns of change* (pp. 29–66). New York: Guilford Press.

Robinson, A., & Elliott, R. (2017). Emotion-focused therapy for clients with autistic process. *Person-Centered and Experiential Psychotherapies, 16*, 215–235.

Rogers, C. R. (1951). *Client-centered therapy*. Boston, MA: Houghton Mifflin.

Rogers, C. R. (1957). The necessary and sufficient conditions of therapeutic personality change. *Journal of Consulting Psychology, 21*, 95–103.

Rogers, C. R. (1959). A theory of therapy, personality, and interpersonal relationships as developed in the client-centered framework. In S. Koch (Ed.), *Psychology: The study of a science* (Vol. 3, pp. 184–256). New York: McGraw-Hill.

Rogers, C. R. (1961). *On becoming a person*. Boston, MA: Houghton Mifflin.

Roth, A. D., Hill, A., & Pilling, S. (2009). *The competences required to deliver effective humanistic psychological therapies*. Centre for Outcomes Research and Effectiveness, University College London. Available online at: www.ucl.ac.uk/clinical-psychology/CORE/humanistic_framework.htm

Sachse, R. (1990). The influence of processing proposals on the explication process of the client. *Person-Centered-Review, 5*, 321–344.

Safran, J. D., & Muran, J. C. (2000). *Negotiating the therapeutic alliance: A relational treatment guide*. New York: Guilford Press.

Salgado, J., Cunha, C., & Monteiro, M. (2019). Emotion-focused therapy for depression. In L. S. Greenberg & R. N. Goldman (Eds.), *Clinical handbook of emotion-focused therapy* (pp. 293–314). Washington, DC: American Psychological Association.

Sanders, P. (Ed.) (2007). *The Contact Work Primer: A concise, accessible and comprehensive introduction to pre-therapy and the work of Garry Prouty*. Ross-on-Wye, UK: PCCS Books.

Sarbin, T. R. (1989). Emotion as narrative emplotment. In M. J. Packer & R. B. Addison (Eds.), *Entering the circle: Hermeneutic investigation in psychology* (pp. 185–201). Albany, NY: State University of New York Press.

Schneider, K. J., & Krug, O. T. (2017). *Existential-humanistic therapy* (2nd ed.). Washington, DC: American Psychological Association.

Shamay-Tsoory, S. (2009). Empathic processing: Its cognitive and affective dimensions and neuroanatomical basis. In J. Decety & W. Ickes (Eds.), *The social neuroscience of empathy* (pp. 215–232). Cambridge, MA: MIT Press.

Sommerbeck, L. (2012). Being nondirective in directive settings. *Person-Centered & Experiential Psychotherapies, 11*, 173–189.

Spinelli, E. (1989). *The interpreted world: An introduction to phenomenological psychology*. London: Sage.

Sutherland, O., Peräkylä, A., & Elliott, R. (2014). Conversation analysis of the two-chair self-soothing task in emotion-focused therapy. *Psychotherapy Research*. Advance online publication. DOI: 10.1080/10503307.2014.885146

Thompson, S., & Girz, L. (2020). Overcoming shame and aloneness: Emotion-focused group therapy for self-criticism. *Person-Centered & Experiential Psychotherapies, 19*(1), 1–11.

Timulak, L. (2015). *Transforming emotional pain in psychotherapy: An emotion-focused approach.* Hove, East Sussex: Routledge.

Timulak, L., & Elliott, R. (2003). Empowerment events in process-experiential psychotherapy of depression: A qualitative analysis. *Psychotherapy Research, 13,* 443–460.

Timulak, L., Iwakabe, S., & Elliott, R. (2019). Clinical implications of research on emotion-focused therapy. In L. S. Greenberg & R. Goldman (Eds.), *Clinical handbook of emotion-focused therapy* (pp. 93–109). Washington, DC: American Psychological Association.

Timulak, L., Keogh, D., McElvaney, J., Schmitt, S., Hession, N., Timulakova, K., Jennings, C., & Ward, F. (2020). Emotion-focused therapy as a transdiagnostic treatment for depression, anxiety and related disorders: Protocol for an initial feasibility randomised control trial. *HRB Open Research, 3,* 7. https://doi.org/10.12688/hrbopenres.12993.1

Timulak, L., & McElvaney, J. (2017). *Transforming generalized anxiety: An emotion-focused approach.* Hove, East Sussex: Routledge.

Warwar, S. H., & Ellison, J. (2019). Emotion coaching in action: Experiential teaching, homework, and consolidating change. In L. S. Greenberg & R. N. Goldman (Eds.), *Clinical handbook of emotion-focused therapy* (pp. 261–289). Washington, DC: American Psychological Association. https://doi.org/10.1037/0000112-012

Watson, J. C., Goldman, R., & Greenberg, L. S. (2007). *Case studies in emotion-focused therapy for depression.* Washington, DC: American Psychological Association.

Watson, J. C., Gordon, L. B., Stermac, L., Kalogerakos, F., & Steckley, P. (2003). Comparing the effectiveness of process-experiential with cognitive-behavioral psychotherapy in the treatment of depression. *Journal of Consulting and Clinical Psychology, 71,* 773–781.

Watson, J. C., & Greenberg, L. S. (2017). *Emotion-focused therapy for generalized anxiety.* Washington, DC: American Psychological Association.

Watson, J. C., & Rennie, D. (1994). A qualitative analysis of clients' reports of their subjective experience while exploring problematic reactions in therapy. *Journal of Counseling Psychology, 41,* 500–509.

Wexler, D. A., & Rice, L. N. (1974). *Innovations in client centered therapy.* New York: Wiley.

Yalom, I. D. (1980). *Existential psychotherapy.* New York: Basic Books.

Zajonc, R. B. (1980). Feeling and thinking: Preferences need no inferences. *American Psychologist, 35,* 151–175.

Index

Tables and Figures are indicated by page numbers in bold print. The letter "b" after a page number stands for bibliographical information in an end-of-chapter "Reading" section.